RUSSELL POTTER & DR. MAITE BALDA

NEW ENERGIZED YOU

How to Feel More Energy and Less Fatigue, According to Science

New Energized You
Russell Potter & Dr Maite Balda
Two Worlds Publishing
www.newenergizedyou.com

New Energized You
Russell Potter & Dr Maite Balda
Published by Two Worlds Publishing
© 2018 Russell Potter & Dr Maite Balda
All rights reserved. No portion of this book may be reproduced in any form without permission from the publisher, except as permitted by U.S. copyright law. For permissions contact:
info@newenergizedyou.com www.newenergizedyou.com
ISBN: 978-1-91643-284-0

The information provided within this book is for general informational purposes only.

While we try to keep the information up-to-date and correct, there are no representations or warranties, express or implied, about the completeness, accuracy, reliability, suitability or availability with respect to the information, products, services, or related graphics contained in this book for any purpose.

Any use of this information is at your own risk.

The methods describe within this book are the author's personal thoughts. They are not intended to be a definitive set of instructions.

The authors recommend speaking with your healthcare professional for items relating to medical health both physical and mental, prior to applying the methods contained within this book.

To those who wish to live a life extraordinary

CONTENTS

Foreword	i
Introduction	1
The Energy Quadrants	1
Bioenergetics	**9**
Where does Energy come from?	9
Glucose's Travels	12
Nutrients and the Brain	19
Oxygen	20
Why does the Brain use so much Energy?	22
Bio Hack 1 | Mitochondrial Biogenesis	25
Bio Hack 2 | Hydration	27
Bio Hack 3 | Cerebral Blood Flow	31
Bio Hack 4 | N4 Sleep	34
Bio Hack 5 | Circadian Rhythm	44
Bio Hack 6 | Diet Hacks	52
Neurological Energy	**73**
Histamine	77
Orexin	80
Orexin Hack | Self-Coaching Before Bedtime	82
Serotonin	90
Serotonin Hack | Sunlight and Pleasant Memories	93
Dopamine	95
Dopamine Hack | Mastering the Short-Term Goal/Reward Cycle	96
Adrenaline and Noradrenaline	97
Adrenaline Hack (Decrease) | Re-perceive Stress as a Friend	99
Adrenaline Hack (Increase) | Put Yourself in Stretch	101
Brain-Derived Neurotrophic Factor	102
BDNF Hack | Complex Movement Cardio	104

Ghrelin	107
Neuro Hack 5 | Stimulants	109

Motivational Energy — 117

Motivation Hack 1 | Challenge your Beliefs: Why You Don't Achieve Your Goals.	122
Motivation Hack 2 | Cognitive Consonance and Value – Goal – Action Alignment	125
Motivation Hack 3 | Positive Psychology	131
Motivation Hack 4 | Locus of Control	139
Motivation Hack 5 | Visualization	141

Energy Efficiency and Environment — 149

Concentration, Flow and Mindfulness	150
How Distraction Saps your Energy	153
Efficiency Hack 1 | Pink Noise or Earplugs	158
Efficiency Hack 3 | Work to a Timer	166
Efficiency Hack 4 | Tracking	169
Efficiency Hack 5 | Task Switching	178
Efficiency Hack 6 | Pause and Restore	179

Conclusion — 193

Acknowledgments	197
About the Authors	199
References	201

FOREWORD

Once in a while you come across a person who has an inexhaustible amount of energy. Inspired, and seemingly with no need for sleep, they can work for extended periods at a high pace with great enthusiasm and joy, never to tire. These people fascinate us, but how do they pull it off? What's their secret

I wrote this book to answer that question.

I've always worked from the desire to help good people to do great things. This has been my guiding light, my compass for over 25 years. To this end, I've been in the business of motivation my whole career, first in the world of talent management, and later in my career, as an author, trainer and executive coach. The aim of talent management is to motivate large groups of people, the aim of coaching is to bring out the best in each person, one at a time. The goal, however, is always the same: to supercharge their motivation and personal energy.

I work with global brands and executives and I love my job. I love seeing people become energized through self-discovery and inspiration. I'm good at my job, but, for years, I knew I had only half of the story. Something was missing. I'd read every bloated and padded book on goals, management, leadership and motivation on the market, but somehow, they just didn't seem to fit with the lives of regular people.

I felt for the corporate people that I trained. They worked hard, very hard, yet at the end of each day, they went home exhausted. In Japan, where I now live, it's common to see people sleeping on their way to work, even on the train platforms. Many Japanese companies have been forced to take extreme action. Some offices now even have lights out at 8pm each day to prevent employees from overworking. The family and personal lives of employees suffer from this continuous fatigue and the problem is not limited to only Japan, this is a global issue.

In life, time is the most precious resource that we have. The passing of my mother many years ago had bought the inevitability of the countdown sharply and viscerally bought that fact into focus. It was no longer television drama, this was real. The valuable lesson I took from that awakening was that we must live every minute with maximum happiness and vitality.

In 2005 I became an entrepreneur. From a successful career in human resources management, I had the dream opportunity to move to a tropical paradise in Asia where I was able to incorporate my own consulting firm, serving startups to global brands. As with most new business owners I was excited and determined, full of the possibilities and eager to make my mark.

Any new entrepreneur will pick up books and read extensively about starting a business. Inevitably, attention will move towards the famous entrepreneurs, those who have trodden the path with great success. We will read the biographies of Branson, Gates, Tony Robbins and the like, and arrive at the conclusion that it takes superhuman levels of energy and focus to get a new business off the ground. And, they'd be right. Throwing yourself on the proverbial grenade in commitment to your new venture is expected, and working marathon hours while maintaining high levels of positive energy is considered the evidence of admonishing oneself to the said grenade.

Having studied the great entrepreneurs as well as top athletes and winners, I noticed that they had one thing in common, hard work, defined as marathon hours of highly productive high paced determined toil, performed for years on end, despite setback after setback before finally….and satisfyingly…breaking though.

When I started my business, I quickly realized that I could work 16-hours per day, fueled on adrenaline, screaming "Geronimo" and boasting of getting just 3-hours of sleep as if it were a badge of honor. The problem was that it simply didn't work. Hard fought gains from the previous days were wiped out as my productivity plummeted. Worse, the adrenaline that fueled me made me confused, anxious and dumb. At times when I needed sharp rational thought, my mind felt like it was full of treacle, slow, foggy and viscous. The highly productive hours were followed by days of low effectiveness as my tired brain simply could not think straight. Mistakes were made, frustrations rose and my enthusiasm waned. How did Bill manage 16-hours per day for 5 years? I wanted to know more. I *needed* to know.

I enrolled my trusty team to help. At each team meeting for the next 3-weeks, each person would bring with them the story of a winner. The tales of wold champions and billionaire legends were recounted at each team meeting. To begin with it was a Wikipedia-fest with clichés and sanitized tales, carefully pressed and released by the well-paid publicists for the protagonists. I was not satisfied. I sent the team back each time to look more deeply. "They weren't born winners, they were made winners, how did this happen?"

As the sessions unfolded the answers became apparent for one subset of super performers in the business world. Childhood events were pivotal. In many, traumatic events had forged incredible fortitude, activating a survival response which would carry them to adulthood success. Forced out of his house at knife point by his mother, Tony Robbins, for example, had to survive alone. The event forced him to survive and eventually to succeed. Conversely, Sir Richard Branson enjoyed the loving parenting of a mother and father who actively encouraged his entrepreneurial skill in an environment where mistakes were welcomed as "The growing pains of an entrepreneur." These were the superstars, but was this true for all successful entrepreneurs?

To find out, I began to interview successful entrepreneurs in Indonesia and Japan. As the interviews developed, almost without exception, a childhood story was revealed; A family in financial trouble, the survival instinct activated, and a highly energized response that continued into adulthood. A father no longer able to work due to illness and a mother forced to work 2 jobs to make ends meet, the child gallantly tries to save the family with their piggy bank.

Many children grow up in traumatic environments that can lead to unfortunate outcomes both immediately and later in life. Instead of being motivated by the survival response, insecurity and self-doubt pervade, and depression and anxiety become major players in their lives, demons to be endured. As I delved further still, the stories unfolded. Each of the successful entrepreneurs had a fateful encounter, a crossroads that would move their fate towards success and away from adversity. Those encounters were with humanity.

Take the tale of a highly successful female entrepreneur who had the energy of a power plant, working long hours at the frantic pace one would expect of a New Yorker, which indeed she was. Abandoned by her parents, she was unfortunate enough to end up in a French orphanage with her younger sister. With no money and no hope, the sisters were destined to walk a difficult emotional path. Distrusting of society and viewing people as selfish, the survival instinct was there but devoid of any hope of ever actually succeeding in life. Then, by luck, they encountered humanity.

An old man, with no interest other than to exercise his deeply held value of compassion, took them under his wing. Not a wealthy man, he bought them clothes and food, even when he had no money for himself. Encouraged by the humanity of the kind man, the sister's already active survival instincts gained the optimistic edge that only hope and humanity can forge, pushing them both to a brighter future. Anything was possible, and indeed, so it proved to be. Now a wildly successful fashion entrepreneur she earns a million-dollar salary and is driven for more. The old man and his wife still visit her once every year.

So, it was clear, you needed childhood trauma and a brush with humanity, or wealthy and very well-adjusted parents to get the wild amounts of focused energy needed to win big in business. I had no hope! Yet, I did possess one thing in great abundance. Curiosity.

I had been looking for the answer to energy and fatigue, but I had fail to ask the question, what is human energy? The answer, I was sure, lay in neuroscience?

I set about the task to discover how the brain uses energy. I uncovered 1000s pages of empirical research papers on neuroscience that began to open the lid on the inner workings of the brain, and how the it utilizes neurotransmitters such as serotonin, dopamine, orexin and histamine to elicit real physical and emotional response. I'm not a neuroscientist, and I initially found the research papers a struggle to comprehend yet truly enlightening. I scoured the pages to find the one nugget that firstly, I could understand, and secondly, would be a vital clue to the solution.

The magic of the brain is that it's really not magic at all, merely an elegant and beautifully evolved chemical-electrical processing organism which can pull any string, emotional or physical, with a sequence of chemical signals. The elegant organism, it seemed, was made for just one thing, survival, and it does this very well indeed. But is there more to it?

Evolution has crafted the brain over hundreds of thousands of years to be fit for purpose. This opens up some beautiful philosophical questions about the nature of man why, indeed, we are here. The notion that we are here simply to eat and reproduce could be a touch simplistic if we look at some of the output of the brain's many systems. Why do we feel great when we see a blue sky and a sandy beach for example?

It also became clear from the research, that as we have become more civilized as a species, we had started to hijack, or hack, the survival systems for non-survival purposes. Take the commercial food industry for example, who use the famous fat, salt and sugar ratio to hijack your serotonin and dopamine systems to make you buy their product again and again. Eating potato chips is no survival activity, in fact its arguably the opposite, yet our systems have been deliberately hacked for the profit of the organization. It really is that simple.

We will explain in detail later in the book how the dopamine system is responsible for one area of energy and motivation called learned behaviors. If major corporations can hack our brains for money, I realized that there was every chance that we could hack our own brains to fight fatigue, to feel more energy, vitality and happiness. This was the answer I was looking for. I could see a way that I could, in the absence of childhood factors, massively increase my own energy and be just like Bill, Richard and Tony. If I could crack the code and hack my own brain, I could help thousands of people to do the same, enjoying higher vitality, and never wasting a moment of their precious lives.

I researched and researched for months, gaining hard fought insights from only published research paper. I was determined that there would be no blog-based pseudoscience involved in the project and as the volume of data research grew I realized that I had enough for a training course and even a book. I was also getting great results from the hacks I was using on myself.

Using the insights, I delivered the training course on energy hacking to a global retailer. The feedback from the participants was overwhelming, "We need this!" With encouraging results for my own personal energy, from the training group, as well as my coaching clients, I decided to press on with the research and to put the findings in a book to reach as many people as I possibly could.

I knew that I wanted the book to be the most thorough and scientifically accurate book on human energy and vitality written to date yet accessible, readable and presenting an easy to use framework to improve the lives of thousands of readers. At that point, little did I know that I was only fraction of the way into the full research journey that it was to become thanks to a partnership with a very talented person.

I knew that my readers would deserve my very best, so I decided to stop the project briefly and find a partner to co-write the book with me, and that person needed to be an experienced neuroscientist and writer. It was my very good fortune to meet Dr Maite Balda.

Foreword Dr Maite Balda

Every living thing needs energy. For us humans, energy is infinitely more complex than batteries to a machine. It is common to see advertisements for magic solutions or short-term energy boosts. .

When I was approached to co-author this book, I was ecstatic to be able to unravel the concept of energy in all its mosaic aspects. I had encountered books focused on diet, others on exercise, others in psychology, biology, neuroscience, real science and pseudoscience. Now, this was our chance to put at all together, offering a 360-view of energy to our readers.

As a scientist, I have always found frustrating when research is not properly interpreted as well as when scientific research is not made accessible to broader audiences. With this in mind I started my own consulting firm, NEUBUCO, seeking to translate scientific discoveries and data accurately into information accessible to anyone. "New Energized You" seeks to inform and help you achieve what works best for you. Energy is a challenge for all of us. Society nowadays requires such a great mental load in so many aspects that it is common for any person to feel a need for higher vitality levels. This book offers not only practical information as to how to achieve this, but it is also bids information based on rigorous academic work.

As a mother of six, I have myself struggled in finding the energy to start/end every day, especially when it starts/ends at unexpected times. Between work, family life, house manegenment, personal care socialization, and daily unexpected adventures, 24 hours a day drained me at my fullest. I didn't even get to look forward to resting on the weekends. Weekends almost seemed like double the work. Between unexpected workload that materialized and being a full-time mom, I finished Sunday's exhausted. When Russell and I started writing this book, we each knew tons about our areas of expertise and looked forward to complementing our knowledge and backing it up with cutting-edge science. Coming from a psychology background and having many years of experience in the field of Cognitive Neuroscience research, partnering up with Russell made lots of sense. Fusing our synergies, experiences, and knowledge we have been able to put together a great book that disentangles the reality of what energy is and how we feel vitality. What we didn't really know, was how much it would actually help us personally.

As an author, I found myself rediscovering information I had forgotten, and practicing hacks myself. It was a process of uncovering that with the years my life had change but I hadn't really adjusted my habits. Maybe more than adjusting my habits, I think that I never really took the time to think about how new circumstances required new habits. For example, making sure I had healthy food I could grab in a hurry. Having washed grapes accessible in the fridge, snack nut bags in plain sight and bananas on my table made sure I didn't look any further when I searched for a quick bite. Another example was my daily routine. My mornings are now not commenced by an alarm that goes off, but by one of my kids having a need. Sometimes it's the need to help them clean up an accident, sometimes someone is thirsty or had a nightmare. Anyhow, for a while I woke up jumping into action without taking a second to think: Hey! It's a new day! Let's make the best out of it! A very simple thought, requires little to no time, but it REALLY changes how you react afterwards. I was so busy with life, I didn't take advantage of times I had to really just find inner peace. The practice of having a moment when everything seems in order and instead of reaching out for my phone to check e-mails or messages, take those 3 minutes to take a couple of deep mindful breaths or fill those 3 minutes with positives thoughts about life. This can be done while cooking, while cleaning you email inbox, vacuuming, before going to sleep or just before you start working. There are tons of opportunities throughout our day to optimize our energy levels, it is up to us to seize them.

In the process of writing this book I learned a lot about myself, about what works best for me and how to feel energized and have the vitality to end and start every day with a genuine smile. Of course, there are days where I feel I can take over the world, and there are others where I am not as successful at optimizing my vitality, but it is about always trying. Being aware that feeling energized depends a lot on you, your behavior, your decisions, your habits and about always starting again, knowing that tomorrow you can always do better.

INTRODUCTION

The Energy Quadrants

Let's be clear, when we talk about energy, we aren't only talking about the fuel that stokes the fire. Energy also englobes the subjective feeling of "can do" confidence that encourages you to strive forward and take on the world in that very moment. The interesting thing about feeling energized is that it takes over you in every area of your life. It is not just about enjoying what you do, but tackling life fully charged. Clearly that feeling of energy is the outcome of a highly complex sequence of processes, pathways, responses and underlying factors originating in our mind and body. Our goal in writing this book was to understand those factors and to present them to you, in a simple, easy to follow, but highly effective, framework. In truth, our writing process was a long evolutionary journey of thorough research and personal testing, which we could never have predicted. The outcomes surprised us. The fruits of our determination illustrated that feeling energized is both highly personal and entirely possible, and can be categorized into four distinct categories or quadrants.

Bioenergetics

As you will read in the section, "Bioenergetics," the first quadrant in our matrix, our physical system. It is a highly sequential and exquisitely evolved masterpiece which requires great care to perform at optimal levels for the duration of our lives. We identified a series of hacks based on solid research and put them to work immediately. In many of the neurology based studies referenced in this book, the benefits of specific nutrients and supplementation are proportionate to the general underlying health of the individual. This means that if you're suffering from an illness such as Alzheimer's, liver disease, or even depression, some hacks might not affect you in the same way they would affect someone in a better health. Likewise, if you're a perfectly healthy adult in your mid-20s, the effects of most dietary interventions may be negligible. The metaphorical Ferrari, straight from the showroom probably can't be tuned much further. Any additional tweaks aren't likely to result in huge gains in performance. The poorly maintained family sedan on the other hand, with 20 years of hard labor under the bonnet, and not a service in its dusty logbook, has significant room for improvement with the best motor oils, a performance tune-up and some high-performance modifications. In our experience, the same is true of many dietary factors.

We, the authors, as with most people, appreciate a quick fix to a problem whenever possible. Yet, we are also people swayed by logic and science more than hearsay and lore. Logically, the first step in our journey was to look deeper into the dietary aspects of human energy. Was there a supplement or food that we could eat that would unlock our inner reactor? We took a closer look at the very building blocks of energy and how our bodies convert the food that we eat into energy. After all, it's what we eat that powers our muscles and brain. We traced the immense journey of glucose, the most important component in the human energy story, from food, through the body's many organs and cells and all the way to the brain.

There is little doubt that the foundations of our subjective energy and vitality sits on the bedrock of good general health and we discuss the most important aspects for energy and vitality in the section.

Neurological

Vitality is perceived in the brain and not merely based solely on our underlying physical health. Given our professional expertise, this was a natural next port of call.

We explored in great depth the elegant dance of neurotransmitters as they relate to vitality and wakefulness, neuron firing, and how their delicate interplay accounts for our feelings of being energized.

The neuroscience quadrant has some of the most important hacks for energy and vitality. Simply understating how to achieve a balance in our neurotransmitter secretion, was an important insight. In our work with training corporations using the Energy Curve, that you will learn about later in this book, many leaders pointed out that their team members had too little energy and needed more adrenaline, whilst they themselves often had too much energy and operated in the unproductive "stress zone." Both groups needed more balance in their mix of neurotransmitter activity in order to be productive.

Ultimately however, we knew that we wanted to control our energy levels on demand, and we assumed that you, the reader, would too. Our experience however, was that stimulating or suppressing neurotransmitters was tough to pull off. The firing of neurotransmitters is a response to many other factors over which we have limited control, including environmental factors such as noise, and learned behaviors and motivators such as fear. We knew that to get the complete picture, we needed to explore both motivation and environment as their own separate quadrants.

Motivational

Think about a time in your life that you felt truly alive, engaged and energized. Maybe you were doing something that meant a lot to you, maybe something that you enjoyed greatly, or maybe you were just working to get something you desperately wanted. In essence, you were motivated.

Our motivators are deeply personal, and they influence our behaviors and emotions profoundly. Clearly, if you know what motivates you, you have arguably the most powerful information in your energy toolkit to feel more vitality and to feel more alive. The challenge, is that most of us are totally unaware of what motivates us. Thankfully for us, however, motivation is one of the most well researched areas of psychology.

There are many continuously evolving theories improving our understanding of motivation, the spark that ignites the neurological cascade of serotonin, dopamine, endorphins and adrenaline. Importantly for us, most motivation techniques are rooted in solid research and time-tested practice. Most are easy to apply and also highly effective for feeling more energy and vitality.

Motivation is fast acting. The intervention you will learn about in the next section, Bioenergetics, are effective within a few days or weeks. The motivation hacks, however, can have immediate impact. As much as we can be motivated to take action, we can also stop ourselves from taking action too. Our beliefs about happiness, energy, vitality, and even success, can stop us from achieving those very things, no matter how much we want them. Feelings of guilt and unworthiness born form our beliefs, for example, can keep us trapped within our comfort zone. Those beliefs are heavy weights that stop us from breaking the surface and gasping the air of our dreams. In the section on Motivation, you will learn how to discover the weights that are holding you under too.

Efficiency & Environment

Focused with laser-like precision on the biological and neurological aspects of the puzzle for so long, we decided to take a step back. We thought long and hard about how more vitality would fit into our day. Where would you find more energy useful and where are you getting fatigued? It took us back to our original motivations for embarking on our journey of discovery into the topic and the two main levels. Firstly, at the experience level, for fully enjoying every minute of life and secondly, the producing level for creating our very best work each day.

At the experience level, we imagined having enough energy at the end of each day or week to pursue interesting new hobbies and doing the things we always wanted to try. From taking up golf to trying amazing new vacation destinations from the bucket list, we imagined living our lives to the fullest. We also imagined having the energy to be enjoyably and genuinely engrossed in fostering relationships.

At the producing and creating level, we imagined writing inspiring texts, musical works or simply just doing the best work of our careers. How could we focus our energy with greater efficiency to produce amazing work and at the same time prevent fatigue? We were naturally curious.

The environmental factor is also hugely important. The very environment that you are in right now has an enormous effect on how you feel emotionally. It can energize you to feel inspired and motivated, or it can sap your energy leaving you fatigued and drained. For example, some of us love to experience the energy of a crowd, others find it exhausting. Some of us do our best work when the environment is silent, while some people prefer to work in group settings with a lot of interaction. The preference is largely down to the person and the situation of course, but at an emotional level, the effect of the environment is indisputable.

The Four Quadrants

We therefore present to you, the four quadrants of our Energy Matrix. Staring with biological energy, the baseline from which you should start your energy hacking journey. We strongly recommend that each and every reader gets a full medical checkup as a starting point. There are myriad underlying medical reasons for feeling low energy which, if diagnosed by a medical professional (and never self-diagnosed from a book or on the internet) there is the real chance of enjoying a dramatic improvement in your energy levels. You may well indeed be the poorly maintained and previously mentioned sedan. Again, the medical checkup is the key. With good health confirmed, we recommend working through the hacks of our first quadrant.

The Energy Zones

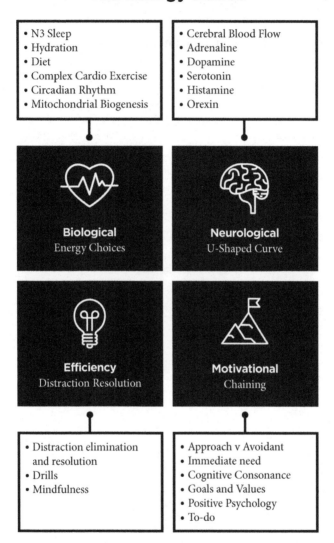

Finding your own formula is key and you may wish to take just one hack from each section to incorporate into your life.

We hope you enjoy hacking your energy in each of the quadrants and encourage you to read each section carefully and to find the right formula for a new energized you.

BIOENERGETICS

Owning the most amazing phone on the market has little to no use if it isn't charged. Any device designed with the best technology available is useless if it doesn't have sufficient energy to function. From the sources of sun, water, wind, fossil or nuclear fuels, transferred efficiently into usable power by generators and engines, all machines rely on a continuous supply of energy and we are no different. Energy is necessary for survival. Every single form of life we know of acquires and transforms energy in order to perform biological work, and humans are no exception. We have the intrinsic need to combine energy sources with oxygen in order to release that energy and to live. No matter how smart or strong we might be, if we are deprived of the most basic elements of water, food or air, we will not be able to thrive. We need a certain amount of energy to think optimally, feel good, and to be energized.

Where does Energy come from?

Energy is the essence of life. Many theories have been proposed to explain the existence of life. In 1949 the big bang theory was developed, explaining that all matter in the universe was originally created from one single point in which all the mass of the universe was concentrated. Due to its high density and temperature, it generated a huge explosion. This massive amount of energy became galaxies, planets, and eventually living beings. That energy, in every sense, created life as we know it.

Stars, for example, run on hydrogen fuel. When stars combine hydrogen atoms to form helium, the star releases heat and light. Eventually a star runs out of hydrogen, its core cools down, and it eventually stops emitting the heat and light. Sometimes collapsing and forming a black hole, sometimes dying slowly over billions of years. A profound and fundamental rule, without energy, there is no life.

In this evolving energy system, humans came to existence. As part of this equation, we are subject to the same energy rules. The main fuel in our system comes from what we eat. Food is our number one source of energy. What we ingest in our daily diet converts into our body's building blocks. The amount of calories we need to consume daily depends on our age, height, weight, and activity level.

Nonetheless, how much we eat is not the only important factor to take into account. *Which* foods we eat, is also fundamental. For example, when we drink milk we get calcium. Calcium is used to build bones, regulate blood pressure, and maintain cell communication. Although some foods are tastier than others, we need a variety of different nutrients to function properly at the end of the day. This is because our body is composed of many different systems, each with different needs.

If you hypothetically dehydrate your brain, most of what is left is fats. In the remaining matter you will also find proteins, amino acids, micronutrients, and glucose. Now, like everything in life, the brain is more than the sum of its individual parts; nonetheless, each one of these components plays a role in the functioning, development, mood, and energy in our bodies. Of the fats in our brain, the superstars are omega-3 and -6. These essential fatty acids, which have been linked to preventing degenerative brain conditions, must come from our diets. Eating omega-rich foods, like nuts, seeds, and fatty fish, is crucial to the creation and maintenance of cell membranes. While omegas are good fats for your brain, long-term consumption of other fats, like trans and saturated fats, might compromise brain health. Not all lipids have the same effect in our body – and this is true with every food group.

Proteins and amino acids are the building blocks of growth and development. They play a significant role in biological processes like oxygen transportation and keeping our immune system healthy. Most of all, proteins are known to be essential for the development of muscles, bones, cartilage, skin, hair, and blood. Proteins also influence how we feel and how we behave. Amino acids contain the precursors for neurotransmitters, the chemical messengers that carry signals between neurons. These affect things like, mood, quality of sleep, attentiveness, and weight. They are one of the reasons we might feel calm after eating a large plate of carbohydrates or more alert after a protein-rich meal.

The complex combinations of compounds in food can stimulate the brain to release mood-altering substances like norepinephrine, dopamine, and serotonin. A diet based on a wide range of foods allows us to maintain a balanced combination of brain messengers and allows our mood to be more stable. Although the brain's weight is only 2% of our body weight, it chews up a whopping 20% of our daily energy resources. The brain, however, is the only organ that cannot store its own energy supply. To function properly, it needs to be in tip-top shape and to have access to a constant supply of energy. Most of the brain's fuel comes from carbohydrates that our body digests and converts into glucose. The frontal lobes of the brain are so sensitive to drops in glucose. That's why a change in mental function is one of the first signals of nutrient deficiency.

Assuming that we are getting glucose regularly, how does each specific type of carbohydrate affect our brain? Carbs come in three forms: starches, sugars, and fibers. While on most nutrition labels they are estimated as one single carb count, the different types act differently within our body. High-glycemic foods, such as white rice, can cause a rapid increase of glucose into the bloodstream and then produces a dip. Blood sugar shoots down, and with it our attention span and mood. On the other hand, oats, grains, and legumes release glucose more slowly, allowing a steadier level of attentiveness.

Following these same principles, nutrients are digested and distributed throughout the body according to the needs of each system and organ. We will look more closely at the nutrition based hacks later in this chapter, and throughout this book.

Glucose's Travels

Glucose, the stuff that powers our muscles to run marathons and our brains to compose concertos, is a traveler on a journey of epic proportions. The journey starts as food and, through hundreds of twists and turns along an ancient and well-trodden path, finally ends at its tiny cellular destination where the magic really happens.

After we swallow our food, acids act on the pulverized package of potential fuel. Enzymes break it down further into a thick sticky liquid called chyme. It's worth noting that without the layer of mucus protecting our stomach, the level of acidity of our gastric juices would easily damage the stomach wall. The fuel package now moves towards the small intestine. It is here where food is broken into molecules, including the all-important glucose. This is how chyme is absorbed into the bloodstream and delivered throughout the body.

From the small intestine, the monosaccharides, including glucose, go directly to the liver, where they are processed. The liver turns any non-glucose sugars, such as lactose, into either glucose or glycogen. The body performs a delicate balancing act where it tries to keep the amount of available glucose to around 4-5 millimoles per liter (mmol/L). Insulin is of key importance here. The primary function of insulin is the regulation of glucose levels in the bloodstream. After a meal, sugar levels rise and insulin is released into the bloodstream. Insulin triggers cells to absorb this sugar and to use it as an energy source.

If you ingest more sugar than your cells need, the multifunctional and very important liver transforms it into storage grade glucose called glycogen,[1] some of which is kept in the liver and the rest of which is stored away in your fat cells until needed. In other words, glycogen is basically glucose that the body can store, whilst glucose continues on through the bloodstream to be taken up by tissues and cells to be used for energy. Given our organs' reserve of glycogen, an average human is able to live an average of three weeks without any food ingestion. There is a different timeline for lack of water ingestion – but we will cross that bridge later.

When glucose levels become lower, a hormone produced in the pancreas tells the liver that the body needs more fuel and that it better start turning some of the stored glycogen back into glucose, or even start using the amino acids for fuel instead.

This whole process is a delightful balancing act that stresses the importance of the pancreas for our energy. The liver, also a vital organ, can store about 100 grams (g) of glycogen and the muscles can store around 400-500 g. This is about enough to get by between meals, and anything extra is stored as fat. In fact, the liver, carries out an estimated 500 functions. For example, it makes bile, which is essential for neutralizing acidic stomach juices and breaking down lipid fats and is therefore crucial in maintaining our energy levels.

When it comes to energy, one of the liver's most important functions is to release glucose into the bloodstream when required. It can do this in three ways:

1. By releasing recently digested glucose.
2. By converting glycogen back to glucose
3. By converting amino acids to glucose . This will only happen if we are fasting.

The liver is our body's gas tank and is extremely important for our energy regulation. It is clear that a healthy liver and pancreas are vital to maintaining high energy levels and avoiding fatigue. The liver is, however, rather easily damaged by an excess of fructose, alcohol.[2][3][4] Controlling our intake of these substances is an obvious hack. Drinking lots of water is the second-best way to care for your liver.

A quick pause here to discuss alcohol consumption. You're probably already aware of the health risks of drinking too much alcohol. Indeed, we love a glass of wine or beer as much as anyone, so we'll focus on the subject briefly purely because of the impact that alcohol can have on the vital organs that control your energy levels. We tend to assume that health problems are limited to alcoholics and the main health issue to avoid is the addiction itself. The truth is a little more complex.

Research defines one drink as either 5oz/148ml of wine (a wine glass typically about a 3rd full), 12oz/360ml of beer (a regular sized bottle or can) or 1.5oz/44ml of spirits (a regular shot). Women who consume 8 or more drinks and men who consume more than 15 drinks per week are clinically considered excessive drinkers.

Excessive alcohol consumption, according to the Center for Disease Control and Prevention (CDC), is responsible for 88,000 deaths per year and costs the U.S. more than $200 billion. More interestingly though, and contrary to what many of us believe, most excessive drinkers are not alcohol dependent. For example, they can go about their lives without craving alcohol and they would not suffer withdrawal symptoms if they stopped drinking. Nonetheless, excessive drinkers are at the highest risk of suffering liver disease or liver cancer regardless of whether they are alcoholics or not. Liver diseases will have huge consequences for your ability to process glucose for energy.

The pancreas is also easily damaged by excessive alcohol intake, something that can eventually lead to pancreatitis.[5] Binge drinking, in particular, is a recipe for disaster.[6] Chronic liver diseases rank as the twelfth most common cause of death worldwide. These disorders are associated with unhealthy lifestyles including excessive alcohol consumption, so it's wise to limit your intake. As a good rule of thumb, drink no more than 2 times a week, and not more than 2 drinks each time.

Luckily, there are also substances that can benefit our organs and boost the way we process energy. Coffee, for example, is a great hack for protecting your liver and, in moderation, is an energy hack. The scientific community has proven over several significant pieces of research that consumption of 1-2 cups of coffee per day significantly reduces the chance of suffering from liver cancer as well as lowering the progression of liver disease.[7] [8] In a nutshell, coffee protects the liver. Coffee has gained even more popularity globally in the past 20 years, and with this increase in consumption more studies are looking into its benefits and possible downsides. It is interesting to know that it is not about caffeine consumption but about coffee itself. Science is still trying to understanding the physiological effects of coffee, but for now, everything seems to point at coffee being able to activate enzymes that detoxify the liver.

Back to our epic journey. Once the liver has helped the glucose to access the bloodstream, it becomes available to other cells. If we are to truly understand how to maximize our energy, we need to understand what happens next.

Once glucose is in the bloodstream and enters a cell, it is not used for fuel in its raw state. Just as petroleum needs to be refined from crude oil, glucose goes through a process too. There is a metabolic reaction that converts glucose into pyruvate and releases adenosine tryptophan triphosphate (ATP), the cell's primary fuel. This form of energy is manufactured inside every cell, in a part called the mitochondria. If you were to look inside a cell, you would find that it looks remarkably similar to an electronic or mechanical device with several working parts, similar to a circuit; only, these ones are made out of organic material.

Mitochondria are essentially the batteries of the cell. They take the glucose and in a lightning-quick process turn it into the all-important ATP. The number of mitochondria in each cell varies, with some cells having just one, and other cells, such as liver cells, having over 2000.[9] What defines how many mitochondria a cell has is its need for ATP. Researches first realized this when they discovered that chickens' breast cells had very few mitochondria compared to pigeons' breast cells. This is because chickens can't fly, while pigeons spend an inordinate amount of time in the air, in addition to being responsible for unique decorative touches to cars and statues all over the world. Pigeon breasts simply need more energy, and therefore more ATP.

Remarkably, the body holds just 250g of ATP at any moment, which is no more than the energy in a single AA battery![10] So, how are we able to run marathons or even get up the stairs with just the power of an AA battery? Well, nature wastes nothing.

Your mitochondria are able to recycle ATP at an incredible rate. Although we have just a small amount of ATP to work with at any given time, just 250g, we actually use around 50-75 kilograms (kg) of ATP everyday. The average adult human goes through their own body weight in ATP each day by recycling it up to 300 times per day. Now that, my friends, is remarkable.

You could imagine that the journey of glucose is like that of a wild salmon returning from the open ocean to the tranquil pools of its birth, covering hundreds of kilometers against a raging river. Once the glucose completes its journey, it powers our brains where our creativity can spawn new and magical experiences and innovations. The final leg of the journey culminates in a truly magical ending.

As we mentioned, glucose can be metabolized and synthesized to ATP. Mitochondria are able to produce energy in the absence of oxygen, although at a much less productive rate. The origins of cellular respiration are so old that even anaerobic organisms, which require no oxygen to grow, are able to transform glucose into ATP. This process is an ancient metabolic pathway that is shared among the vast majority of living organisms. Nonetheless, in humans, mitochondrial performance and energy production thrive with oxygen, and there is a hack to achieve this (which we will come to later).

And so, glucose completes its epic journey. A miraculous and ancient pilgrimage performed every day in each and every one of us. Now you know how energy is made and how it relates to the availability of energy in your body, the next question is how does this apply to your emotional feeling of vitality and positive energy? Does having more mitochondria mean that we can have more energy? Will we simply have more energy if we consume more food?

The answer is no on both counts. The amount of mitochondria that we have does not directly influence the amount of energy that we are able to use. Our brain's and our body's limiting factor is not the amount of mitochondria that we have, but the fine equilibrium between biological processes that influence the brains main systems.

The same applies to food consumption. There are foods that have a high calorie count, but this energetic value does not translate into higher energy. This is due to the fact that food by itself is not fuel – it has to be processed by our body and transformed. This transformation can be more or less optimal depending on the specific qualities of the food including its chemical composition, digestion time, and its vitamin and mineral content. Each digestive process takes a minimum amount of time and bodily effort. For this reason, more food doesn't mean more energy.

In fact, the average human consumes more energy than we are able to use daily. A stick of butter (113g) has 810 calories, contains 290% of saturated fat daily value percentage, and 81% of cholesterol. A cup and a half of kale (100g) has 49 calories, 0% saturated fat and cholesterol, 199% of recommended daily amount (RDA) of vitamin A, and 200% of vitamin C. As you can see, the same amount of food can have a significantly different composition and impact on the body. Our body has no substantial use for highly saturated fats, but it can do wonders with a proper intake of vitamins. Lower calorie foods can supply a higher amount of valuable energy to our body if they have sufficient vitamin and mineral profiles as compared to high calorie foods in general. This is because calories are only a measure of the potential energy stored in the food, but food itself is not made up of calories any more than water is made of milliliters.

Foods with more calories supply your body with more energy per bite, but also take longer to burn. They can also produce an excess of energy that will be placed into fat cells that grow and expand, causing weight gain.

For this reason, it is not about the calorie content of the food, but about its nutrient composition instead.

Nutrients and the Brain

Let's continue the journey of glucose. At this point, we have glucose in our blood and it reaches the blood brain barrier (BBB). The BBB is like a fine sieve that prevents toxins and microorganisms from entering our brain. The BBB was first suggested by Paul Ehrlich and later by Edwin Goldman following their observation that when cell dyes were injected into the bloodstream, specific ones showed up in the brain whilst others didn't.

It's important to remember that ours brains control all bodily functions. It is the conductor of the symphony that is our living, breathing body. Not only does it control movement and hormone secretion, but it is also responsible for our thought process, memory storage, sensory perception, and emotional state of course. Our brain is the keeper of our personality, our identity, and our feeling of vitality and motivation. Being such a vital organ, it makes sense that it has many layers of protection. A hard skull is not the only protection we have against damaging the brain. Our BBB is a filter that allows only glucose, amino acids, and some hormones, such as insulin, to pass through. It is able to prevent large molecules, including most bacteria and viruses, from reaching the delicate tissue of the brain. Although we need a very healthy BBB to have a healthy brain, the downside of the BBB is that it prevents nearly all medications from reaching the brain.[11] Doctors and researchers treating brain related illnesses are constantly seeking ways to allow medications to reach the brain's tissues.

However, the BBB is not infallible. A chronic lack of sleep can put the BBB at risk, as it makes it more permeable. This leaves the brain in a more vulnerable state, specifically in the region of the hippocampus. This is the region where we store memories and where most of our identity is contained.[12] It's very important to know that the BBB is a two-way filter that not only prevents toxins from getting in, it also lets toxins out of the brain too. Getting a great night's sleep is essential for blood brain barrier health and for your energy and vitality and you will learn how to achieve this in the section on N3 Sleep.

Oxygen

Oxygen has become a synonym for both vitality and for life itself. Oxygen is not only in the air we breathe, but also in the water we drink. Almost all living things require oxygen at some level so it's not surprising that oxygen and life are so closely related in the language of popular culture.

Without oxygen, human cells wouldn't be able to release the energy in the foods that we eat. Most brain cells will begin to die after 4-6 minutes without oxygen. What makes our blood so important to us is its role in transporting oxygen around the body.

Oxygen facilitates the breaking down of chemical bonds to release the energy held within. The body uses oxygen, which it cannot store, to release approximately 2,000 calories per day from the food that we consume. Oxygen is vital for our survival but, astoundingly, it actually performs only one task in the entire body. Our bodies are astounding. We often forget that nearly all of the processes that lead to movement, perception, and all of the things that we enjoy, happen at an atomic level. We are a whole lot more than a beating heart and a thinking brain. Indeed, Brett Wagner at the University of Iowa Free Radical and Radiation Unit describes it as, "One of the major developments during evolution… [was the] ability to capture dioxygen in the environment and deliver it to each cell in the multicellular, complex mammalian body ".[13]

Research indicates that our brains use more oxygen when processing cognitively demanding tasks. It seems that the brain also recruits more glucose and blood flow to activated brain regions. In fact, the increase in oxygen is less than the increase in blood flow and glucose to the specific brain area in use. It seems like oxygen supplies the extra energy required, and although essential, it is not the star in cognitive processes. In other words, we need extra oxygen to think, but having extra oxygen won't influence our thought quality. That said, too little oxygen certainly will.

Sipping cans of 100% pure oxygen will not only be ineffective, it can also be dangerous. The reason is that oxygen in high concentrations can be toxic and lead to seizures, especially if the oxygen is at a higher pressure than the atmosphere.[14] Ironically, too much oxygen at atmospheric pressures leads to death by oxygen starvation, as the lungs struggle to cope and shut down because oxygen is vasoconstrictive. Yes, too much oxygen will suffocate you!

Oxygen in high concentrations is also toxic in a cellular level. Cells react badly to oxygen and quickly use up their supplies of antioxidants, as oxygen is highly corrosive. However, the body does have ways to protect its cells from overexposure to oxygen.

Breathing good quality air is a way of getting more from oxygen in a natural and healthy way. That means air with 21% oxygen and no more than regular atmospheric amounts of CO_2, as higher levels of CO_2 displace O_2. This is where it gets tricky – offices and classrooms have higher concentrations of CO_2, so high that they have been shown to make a significant dent in our ability to think properly.

More than that, CO_2 makes you sleepy. The drowsy side effect is the first indication that you could be about to die of CO_2 poisoning. Scientists from University of California, Berkeley have proved that regular office-quality air, which has around 2-3 times higher concentrations of CO_2 than optimal, negatively affected performance in 6 out of 9 tests! Researchers also found that concentrations of CO_2 in meeting rooms and classrooms could be 3 times higher than in regular office space.[56]

The hack here is for the senior managers at organizations to wake up to this issue and to monitor the air quality to ensure that we are actually getting 21% oxygen. Measurement devices are cheap and available online. If air quality is poor, it's a sign that the ventilation or air conditioning is not working properly, or that the density of people is too high, or both.

Breathing air contaminated with high levels of CO_2 and less than 21% oxygen leads to feelings of fatigue and low energy. Most of us don't have the luxury of opening an office window, but taking a walk, leaving meeting room doors open and raising it as an issue with your manager can help. Supplementing oxygen from canisters is not advised however. While oxygen levels around the standard 21% allow for peak cognitive performance, the negative effects of going higher (i.e., free radical damage) by using supplementary oxygen does not warrant the risk.

Why does the Brain use so much Energy?

The brain is a gas guzzler. If it were a car, it would be a Mustang. The brain uses a whopping 20% of all the calories we consume each day, yet it weighs only 2% of our bodymass.

The brain recruits energy in the same way as the other organs of the body. As with liver cells, brain cells have a high level of mitochondria to provide the ATP needed for its functioning. So why does the brain need so much energy?

The answer is very simple, your brain is never off, even when your sleeping, Even at the times we do not process the world through our eyes, our brain takes the available sensory information and reconstructs the reality around us. It is constantly analyzing external as well as internal stimuli.

The brain is always *on* and operating at a very high level, whether we are resting with our eyes shut, admiring a beautiful view, or solving complex equations. Researcher David Atwell and his colleagues from University College London have shown that there is only a 6% increase in energy consumption to activate conscious perception.[15]

This is fundamentally important for our understanding of brain energy. The brain is not a muscle. When we sit down to rest our leg muscles they use very little energy, the brain however uses a lot of energy all of the time.

Each brain cell is always in one of two modes, excited or inhibited. Both states require a lot of energy. You can visualize it as the combined energy of two people engaged in an arm wrestling competition. That, in essence, is how the brain works. It is also crucial to remember that the brain has no way of storing energy.

Despite this, the brain and body are fine-tuned for energy efficiency. It likes to save energy where possible, which explains boredom and fatigue when doing one activity for a long a time. It's trying to get you to rest, use less energy and to recover.

It may be a touch misleading to think that we get tired because of a lack of glucose in the brain. Although that may be true for intense, short muscle workouts (otherwise known as momentary muscle failure), many of you will have experienced that running over longer distances at a slower pace, the body has an incredible amount of energy at its disposal to keep gong for long periods of time. When lifting heavy weights, our muscles quickly run out of ATP, most of which can be replaced in around 30 seconds. With endurance exercise, our muscles can replenish the ATP quickly enough that we can continue without stopping. The brain, it would seem, is more like the endurance athlete and, as we will see in the diet hacks section of this book, it has an emergency backup supply called phosphocreatine, just in case.

The brain is in charge of many functions, and not all require the same amount of energy. The amount of glucose used in a specific brain region depends on the task and also the aptitude, defined as natural ability, of the person. A study from Berkeley concluded that people with high aptitude used more glucose on a difficult test than those with low aptitude.[16] Maybe the low aptitude guys gave up on the test – who's to say? Nonetheless, this does show that when our brain is fully engaged in something within our natural sphere of expertise, our brains seem to light up more due to its need for more oxygen, glucose and blood flow.

Alternatively, fluency of skill, which often follows years of intense training, uses less brain energy. Research for Mount Sinai indicates that, for verbal fluency at least, our brains use less energy when we are more fluent, which indicates that expertise practiced to the point that it requires less cognitive effort is more efficient. This theory opens up the possibility of yet another energy hack. By practicing the tasks and activities you do regularly, to the point that you can do them without thinking, may save your brain precious energy.[17]

Now that we know how our glucose travels from food to cell, how it enters the brain through the blood brain barrier, and why the brain uses so much of it, let's look at some bio hacks which are proven to increase your energy and vitality.

Bio Hack 1 | Mitochondrial Biogenesis

Mitochondrial biogenesis is one of the ways that the body can enjoy more physical energy capacity. It is the process of increasing the number of energy producing mitochondria in our body. The process involves the splitting or fusing of existing mitochondria into new ones, which then enables greater amounts of ATP to be produced for the cell to use.

Increasing the number of mitochondria is analogous to adding an extra engine to an airplane. It should be noted that an airplane with ten engines would be suboptimal, its massive weight and fuel needs would be impractical. The same goes for mitochondria. We should avoid going overboard with any synthetic or artificial multiplication of mitochondria, but there is a benefit in gently increasing the number of mitochondria a little through the natural methods.

Mitochondrial biogenesis is a complex process that involves several hormones and proteins, and the process only happens in certain circumstances. Those circumstances include strenuous exercise (especially endurance), exposure to cold temperatures, and an absence of glucose. The mitochondria receive their orders from a "factor" called PGC-1α (peroxisome-proliferator-activated receptor γ coactivator-1α), which increases the number of mitochondria by splitting them and thereby creating more of them.

The most important neurotransmitter and hormone involved in the regulation of mitochondrial biogenesis is AMPK. Think of AMPK as a type of "energy sensor" within the cell. It is essential for energy metabolism and plays an important role in the brain's learning processes too. When AMPK perceives a lack of energy, it activates PGC-1α, which gives the mitochondria the order to split. Increasing AMPK, it would seem, would be our goal. As we will see later in the book, there are ways to increase AMPK with complex movement cardiovascular exercises.

Research is clear: exercise increases mitochondrial biogenesis in both the brain and skeletal muscle tissues.[18] But researchers also found that by simply increasing AMPK, without exercise, mitochondrial biogenesis was induced.[19] This can be also achieved with exposure to very cold temperatures, such as ice baths or cold water swimming.

AMPK is the actual reason why ice baths or cold water swimming have been linked to longevity factors that have been shown to extend life span in numerous organisms. Apart from producing new mitochondria and reducing fat storage, AMPK increase promotes healthy blood glucose and lipid levels.

If cold water baths don't sound like your thing, there is one training modality in particular which research suggests can increase AMPK. The high-intensity interval training (HIIT), done in hypoxia.[20]

Hypoxic training means starving your body and brain of oxygen with the hope that, when regular oxygen supply is restored, you will feel superhuman and better utilize your oxygen. This approach is often used by elite athletes. You can do this either by flying to Peru, or some other high-altitude location, for an intense workout, by buying a special training mask, or simply by breathing only through your nose during training. There is remarkably little research to support that this increases athletic performance, but lots of significant research that proves this increases AMPK, which can lead to more energy.

Research suggests that in moderately fit (but not elite) athletes there is an up-regulation of mitochondrial biogenesis and mitochondrial density from hypoxic training. Although the jury is out about whether hypoxic training is any better than regular training for general fitness levels, when it comes to the mitochondrial biogenesis, the type of training does have some effect.

For those seeking advanced athletic fitness levels, researchers are keen to point out that although athletes may enjoy more mitochondria and energy, they are also likely to be exercising at suboptimal intensity, which would have given them the performance improvement they were looking for in the first place. If you're an elite athlete looking to increase your mitochondria we suggest the ice or calorie restriction method.

Calorie restriction could be the safest and least painful way to increase your mitochondrial biogenesis. There is evidence that moderate calorie restriction can increase mitochondrial biogenesis and energy efficiency, causing us to use less oxygen without the side effects of oxidative stress.[21] Remember, that more calories does not equate to more usable energy, its where the calories come from that counts.

Bio Hack 2 | Hydration

As Benjamin Franklin once said, "When the well is dry, we know the worth of water." Few, however, know the worth of water when the well is flowing properly.

We know what you're going to say. *Water, really? I paid good money for this book and that's all you can come up with?* As you'll find out shortly, water is so fundamental to energy, and so delightfully elegant in its method, that a whole book could be dedicated to it.

Water is indeed essential for energy. Amongst many other things, it transports nutrients to, and removes waste from, our cells.[22] Water is essential for the use of oxygen and nutrients in all cells.[23] [24] [26]

Water not only composes nearly 60% of our body, but our blood itself is almost 80% water. Blood is responsible for distributing oxygen throughout the body, collecting waste, regulating body temperature, and preventing blood loss through coagulation. The circulatory system and the muscular system work together when we exercise to provide for the increased demands of energy and strength, which increase the blood flow to our muscles. This is also true in the brain. Blood rushes to active brain areas to supply firing neurons with the oxygen and glucose they need for energy. Cerebral blood flow is responsible for getting oxygen and nutrient supplies to the necessary brain areas. In this way, cerebral blood flow is vital for feelings of energy and vitality and for high-performance cognition, which means that the body needs the right volume of blood to begin with. One of the vital roles of water is to help maintain the right volume of blood in the cardiovascular system.[25] In order to provide our brain with a proper level of oxygen, maintaining blood flow is a must.

Dehydration is the enemy. A dry mouth, anxiety, and overheating are only three of the symptoms of dehydration. When fluid output exceeds intake by more than 5%, dehydration is classified as severe. Although severe cases are not common in the general population, moderate dehydration is more common than we might think.

It has been reported that 75% of the population of highly developed countries fall short of consuming the 1.5 liters of water per day recommended by the World Health Organization. This means that most people in these countries are functioning in a chronic state of mild dehydration (1%-2% loss of body water). So you are statistically likely to be dehydrated this very second. When you are hungry you feel it. Your tummy rumbles, and you literally feel faint when your blood glucose level dips. When you get severely dehydrated, your mouth gets dry and your skin gets dried and itchy, but this is not the case for mild dehydration.

The thing with mild dehydration is that it silently decreases your cognitive function and your mood, without an alarming signal to let you know such as a hunger pang or dry mouth.

The main problem with dehydration is that it plays a massive role in both physical and mental performance. Adequate hydration not only prevents the development of disease, but also significantly enhances how alert you feel.[17] Dehydration by heat exposure or exercise has been shown to significantly decrease alertness, concentration, attention, visuomotor tracking performance, and short-term memory.[26][27] It promotes a bad mood, tiredness, headaches, and increased reaction times. Interestingly, studies have shown that dehydration will not affect the amount of correct answers on a test but will affect how long it takes to answer them. In other words, it makes you slower and more lethargic.

Unsurprisingly, studies have also found that the response time was even larger when subjects were both fatigued *and* dehydrated. Male volunteers in this state were given an ominous sounding "six-task cognitive test battery" followed by questionnaires to test how "off" they were feeling. Yes, they actually volunteered for this. The results were clear: mild dehydration induced adverse changes in vigilance and working memory, and increased tension, anxiety, and fatigue.[28] It's the same story for women. In another study by the same group, the researchers found degraded mood, increased perception of task difficulty, lower concentration, and headache symptoms from just minor dehydration in the women tested.[29]

Dehydration has similar effects to a mild concussion, most notably visual memory impairment and fatigue.[30] This is clearly not optimal for vitality. Nobody in their right mind would opt for a mild concussion every day, but by not staying optimally hydrated you are effectively saying, "Hit me!"

It is theorized that the reason for mental impairment may be due to the contraction of blood vessels as the body fights to maintain hydration, possibly through a decrease in blood volume. This, in turn, reduces the flow of oxygen to the brain, which may be the cause of the impaired cognitive function observed by scientists.

Hydrating is one of the simplest yet most effective hacks you could follow. So, how much water should you drink?

We all need, on average, just 1.5 liters (l) per day.[31] That's right, just 1 large bottle. As we often forget to drink when we eat (which is when we need it the most), be sure to grab a large 500 milliliter (ml) glass of water with every meal, and you'll be in the right zone. That takes care of the 1.5l, but when exercising or in more humid climates, consciously drink more throughout the day – or do as Italians do. In Italy, every espresso comes with a glass of water. You can follow that time-honored tradition even if you drink lattes from Starbucks. Just go smaller with the cup size, i.e. downgrade your *venti* to a *grande,* and grab some water too. Less milk is a good choice, as it's very difficult for your liver to convert milk to glucose. You can energy-hack and look sophisticated at the same time.

Essentially, you should drink when you're thirsty, at mealtimes and add more water into your daily routine. Note that alcohol does not count, however, and will in fact significantly impair your hydration. The famous urine color test is a great ally here. If urine is dark yellow in color, you need to drink more water. If it's clear, you're in the right zone. If you're not sure, asking strangers for a second opinion could land you in trouble, and if you're color blind, we can't help you.

As 75% of us, in developed nations, are likely to be dehydrated, staying in your comfort zone with the amount you drink will not work, and you will need to consciously drink more. If you have one of those *I'm-drinking-a-lot-of-water* epiphany moments, you know you're making the change you need to achieve optimal hydration and more energy.

I hope we've made the case for hydration as a vital energy hack. Drinking more water is such a simple one, but we cannot overstate the impact that it has on energy. Sometimes we look for the unknown, the competitive edge that only *we* know about. Conversely, we get fed so much advice through the media about what we should and shouldn't do for our health that it's hard to know what to commit to. In this book you will learn that energy is a very personal pursuit and that there are few one-size-fits-all solutions but water is definitely one of them.

Time and again we have been told to drink water and that the importance of drinking water is paramount to our health. Our bodies are 60% water, people so it may be hard for us to believe that our soft, squishy bodies are in any way short on water but in all likelihood, they almost certainly are. When it comes to brain energy, however – the kind of high-vitality mental energy we desire – hydration really is where it's at.

Bio Hack 3 | Cerebral Blood Flow

More oxygen does not help with enhanced brain performance as much as increasing blood flow and glucose do.[32] Increased blood flow to the brain is the result of the brain's arteries becoming wider, and that's called vasodilation. Vasodilation is the widening of arteries, including those in the brain. This can result in a drop in blood pressure. Although this may seem like a bad idea, studies indicate that, in the brain at least, vasodilation increases cerebral blood flow and has a positive effect on cognition. The brain has an insatiable need for nutrition but can store little energy. As with any other portable machine, the brain is on an energy budget. All successful inventions that have endured the test of time, like clocks, laptops, motorbikes, and jumbo jets, have an internal system to store and efficiently use its energy. The brain gets its energy supply from constant cerebral blood flow.

So how does vasodilation in the brain work? It begins with the cells that make up the lining for the arteries in the body and brain, called endothelial cells. These cells respond to specific chemical signals to either constrict or dilate. The main trigger to dilate is provided by nitric oxide, but there are others including adenosine, adrenaline, L-arginine, histamine, and niacin.

One of the best ways to ensure a specific type of vasodilation, related to having healthy blood vessels, is called flow-mediated vasodilation. This is the extent to which the blood vessels can expand and stretch under the pressures of the blood flow itself. It can be seen as a measure of the health of blood vessels. An excellent way to increase this is by eating omega-3 fatty acids. A number of studies which measured the effects of omega-3s on cerebral blood flow indicated an increase in a wide spectrum of subjects, from smokers to elite athletes.[33]

A review of the significant number of studies of the supplement showed moderate positive effects on the healthy functioning of arteries in healthy people, whilst the effect on those with chronic diseases was even more significant.[48]

As is often the case with research that appears to give great hope, the subsequent studies can often be a little disappointing and due to the limitations in the design of the research. This often relates to the range of test subjects available for each study. Many studies use university students as a useful controlled group, as opposed to people from a wide range of age profiles and situations. In this book, we give you the proven facts and also we also share our own opinions based on observation and experience and our knowledge of studies in the field.

To date, there has been no study which has conclusively proved the link between increased vasodilation, cerebral blood flow and cognitive performance. One study involving students showed clear evidence of increased cerebral blood flow in the prefrontal cortex (PFC), however they found no significant improvement in cognitive performance. As university students are already at their mental prime, logically the effects could be limited. Many other studies have shown significant cognitive improvement in people with impaired cognitive function after supplementation with omega oils.[34][35]

We suggest that for the average person, increasing cerebral blood flow is an energy hack. We can tell you personally that a one-minute running-on-the-spot routine is enough to give the writers of this book a potent shot of mental energy, and we use this in training workshops as an icebreaker to energize otherwise lethargic participants..

Cerebral blood flow has other compensatory functions in the brain, which auto-regulates it and compensates for decreases in oxygen and nutrition by increasing the volume of blood flowing through. Researchers studied a large group of older adults at high risk for developing Alzheimer's Disease (AD). Adults with risk of developing AD have a high amount of amyloid beta in their brain. This results in a huge increase in blood flow. Interestingly enough, when their cognitive performance was compared to a control group, no significant difference was found. This means that the brain is actually increasing blood flow to compensate for the neuronal death in areas associated with AD.[36] Based on this large study, adequate cerebral blood flow is clearly vital for brain functioning and, of course cognitive performance.

So, other than a healthy supply of Omega 3 oils and exercise, how else can you ensure proper cerebral blood flow?

In the Diet Hacks section of this chapter we will show you which foods are proven to support stronger cerebral blood flow in credible research, but as a teaser for now, research has found a positive correlation between Vitamin D and brain blood flow.

Another way to increase cerebral blood flow is with brain exercises. Some of the most successful techniques include meditation, dedicating 30-minutes a day to thinking about goals and ways to improve yourself, contemplating things you are grateful for, mindfulness, or even prayer can significantly enhance cerebral blood flow as studies have show. In the final chapter of the book you will learn more techniques that will help you to maintain not only enhanced cerebral blood flow but also focus, allowing you to use your hard earned energy with more efficiency.

In conclusion, cerebral blood flow is an excellent energy hack for a healthy brain, fighting fatigue and increased vitality. As the brain can't store energy, the additional nutrition, especially glucose, is just what you need for more mental energy.

Bio Hack 4 | N3 Sleep

Not in vain do we spend one third of our lives sleeping. Sleep is not only vital for survival but is also one of the most neglected needs of our time. Let's imagine that our brain is a car, which, like most machines, requires fuel for energy and, if not regularly serviced and repaired, will eventually break down (usually on a rainy day with the kids in the back). The brain, like any car, requires regular maintenance. As luck would have it, evolution has provided built-in mechanisms to self-maintain. The only catch is that this only happens when we sleep.[37]

Dolphins and birds are able to keep half their brain asleep while the other half is awake. Humans, alas, are not able to pull this off. The very fact that we need 8 hours of sleep puts us humans in an extremely vulnerable position for predation, evolutionarily speaking. Not only do we spent 8 hours unconscious having occasional vivid hallucinations i.e. dreaming, but many natural human predators are actually nocturnal.

As we lie happily in bed at night, an incredible process of neuronal cleaning takes place which effectively washes and services the brain. You may at first think that you can learn without sleep, and to some degree, yes, you can. But for long-term retention, sleep does wonders, and it requires no cost, effort, or additional total time devoted to study sessions. Sleeping provides optimal conditions for processes that integrate newly encoded memory into long-term storage. Memories are reactivated during sleep, when new memories that are prone to decay are transformed into stable memories that are preserved for the long-term.[38] Sleep not only helps to strengthen memories, but also to actively forget irrelevant information, thus optimizing memory for what is relevant.[39]

Rapid Eye Movement (REM) sleep, which comes at the end of a full sleep cycle, is thought to play an active role in learning by integrating newly encoded memories with pre-existing knowledge. [40]

If we fail to get enough sleep, our poorly maintained brain begins to resemble next doors' rusty station wagon rather than the purring Ferrari we're after. This is quite literally the case, as the tired brain endures an increase in damaging oxygen reactive species (ORS), i.e., the same stuff that rusts cars and also damages our cells. Sleep deprivation can cause serious mental impairment in decision making, cognition, and of course energy. That very fact was indeed the reason that this book came to be.

A chronic lack of sleep can have irreversible effects on our brains. That's right, irreversible. With just three hours less sleep than we need, the mitochondria in our brains fight back with a release of an antioxidant called SirT3. The fact that it is releasing an antioxidant is a sure indicator that the brain is protecting itself from the effects of sleep deprivation. More disturbing, however, is the effect of severe sleep loss, which means losing all 8 hours of sleep per day. In this extreme circumstance, SirT3 is completely stopped, however, the ROS (the damaging free radical inducing compounds) are actually increased. In effect, this means that the brain has given up the fight. Researchers have found that this can cause irreversible damage to neurons, specifically their mitochondria which are vital for energy.[41]

Although we know that most readers will rarely lose an entire night's sleep, there are undoubtedly times when we will go several nights with drastically reduced snooze time.

It's worth remembering that although the brain gets all of its glucose and oxygen from the blood supply, the ATP derived from glucose, which powers the brain, is produced in the mitochondria of brain cells.

A study involving over 20 medical organizations in the U.S. concluded in their report, published by the Sleep Foundation, that for an adult between the ages of 26 and 64, 7-9 hours' sleep is optimal, with 6 hours being the lower limit and 10 the upper limit.

The study showed that worryingly, when we are sleep deprived, we may be completely unaware that our cognition has been impaired. Further, it seems that it is the *length of wakefulness*, rather than the lack of sleep, that is the main determinant of our cognitive performance. In other words, trying to get in 12 hours of sleep and then expecting to pull off a 2-day wakeful marathon will not work.

People who sleep 4-6 hours during 14 consecutive nights perform as if they had endured sleep deprivation of 2 days. The only difference between these people and the 48-hour sleep deprivation group is that the people who sleep 4-6 hours for 14 days report their cognitive productivity as normal. Short-term sleep deprivation produces global decreases in brain activity. The larger reductions are found in the distributed cortico-thalamic network which controls attention and higher-order cognitive processes. It has been observed that people who sleep 4-6 hours for 7 days straight take longer than 3 days to return to their baseline efficiency and productivity.

Researchers at the University of California, San Francisco discovered that some people have a gene that enables them to do well on 6 hours of sleep per night. This gene, however, is very rare, appearing in less than 3% of the population. For the other 97% of us, 6 hours doesn't come close to cutting it.

We rely on our cognitive functions to make decisions, but sleep loss has the same effect as mild alcohol intoxication. Drunk drivers will step into their car believing that they can drive perfectly well when it is clearly not the case. Sleep deprivation has the same effect, in both impaired judgment and impaired skill. The road haulage industry has known this for years, which is why they impose limits on the amount of time a truck driver can drive without getting sleep.[42]

Going 17 hours without sleep is comparable to having a 0.05% blood alcohol level. This means that if you wake up at 6am, by 11pm you are functioning with impairment in reflexes, reasoning, depth perception, peripheral vision, glare recovery, concentration, reaction time, gross motor control, and judgment. Superman never saved Metropolis under the effects of alcohol, nor did Batman ever rescue Gotham City while legally drunk. As with superheroes, a good professional would never work under the influence, not only because it would be socially reproachable, but because it would be an invitation for mistakes. Yes, it is true that sometimes work requires intense periods of labor: a deadline, a drastic change of direction, or any other need. Nevertheless, being awake for 21 hours is comparable to a blood alcohol level of 0.08%.

Cutting our sleep short has consequences for neuron health, cognitive performance, reaction times, neural repair, energy, removing neurotoxins, and of course our feeling of vitality. Let's remind ourselves that sleep deprivation damages the mitochondria, which is where our energy is actually produced, and orexinergic cells, which are essential for keeping us awake.

Sleep can be split into two parts: NREM (Non-Rapid Eye Movement) and REM (Rapid Eye Movement). REM is sometimes referred to as "paradoxical sleep," because in this light sleep state, our brain's electrical activity looks a lot like when we are awake and deeply relaxed. We cycle in and out of each phase 3 to 4 times throughout the night.

Sleep is further split into four more distinct phases: the bit at the beginning when you snooze off (N1), the bit where your muscles become incapacitated and you may have a waking dream (N2), and a deeper phase of sleep (N3) where the rock and roll happens. The final phase (N4) is the deepest sleep state.[43]

Crucially, one specific phase of our sleep, the N3 sleep phase, is the restorative phase when tissues are repaired, memories are processed, and energy is restored. The N3 phase is crucial for growth, neuroplasticity, neuronal cleaning, and energy replenishment.

However, this phase lasts for only 3-4 minutes, and this time reduces as we get older.

Unless the brain removes neurotoxic substances, its working efficiency in terms of real energy and subjective fatigue is significantly affected. In fact, as we mentioned earlier in the book, the blood brain barrier (BBB) exists for the purpose of *preventing* neurotoxins and pathogens such as bacteria from entering the brain. A lack of sleep makes the BBB more porous, which allows toxins in, compounding the problem. One can imagine that some of the effects that we feel after diminished sleep are due to a toxic event in the brain induced by a leaky, sleepy BBB and insufficient time in clearing our neurotoxic waste.

Some of the neurotoxins that are cleared during sleep can cause a lot of damage if left in the brain. One of the most damaging is beta amyloid, which is a byproduct of metabolism and is associated with Alzheimer's disease. Beta amyloid is not the only neurotoxic waste that's cleaned while we sleep, but it is perhaps the most important.

Understanding the process for clearing neurotoxic waste is important for realizing the importance of quality sleep.[44] So, how does the brain pull off this feat of neuronal cleaning, and why does it only happen when we sleep?

Researchers found that when we sleep, there is a 60% increase in the space around brain cells which hold cerebrospinal fluid, and for a very good reason. The increase in space allows convection processes in the fluid to remove the neurotoxic waste. Again, this only happens when we sleep, so getting 7-9 hours of sleep and reaching the N3 sleep phase is vital. This means that the sleep must be uninterrupted – and the quality of sleep is key. All of the hacks later in this section are about maintaining high-quality sleep, and this should be your goal.

Purely in terms of energy expenditure, the longer we stay awake, the more energy our brains consume. Specifically, it's the rate of energy use that increases. It's akin to starting a journey in a car with a fuel consumption of 30 miles per gallon (mpg) and arriving at the destination with the same car guzzling gas at 10mpg. Remember, it's the length of wakefulness that counts.[45]

It's a clear warning to us. A higher ATP production increases the oxidative stress on cells, which can lead to cell damage without antioxidant protection. Taken together, this is the strongest argument against marathon sessions of wakefulness for feelings of energy and vitality.

We know you get the picture by now, and we promised that by the end of the chapter you would look at sleep somewhat differently. So, how to hack the perfect night' sleep?

Optimize the Sleeping Conditions in your Room.

One of the most important sleep hacks is the room itself. For quality, grade-A sleep, the room you sleep in must be both dark and silent. Having light impacting your closed eyelids can disturb your sleep, so making sure the room is moderately dark is essential. Sound is also important, and the *ping!* of your social media app is enough to break your sleep cycle and interrupt your crucial energy renewal.

If it's not possible to cut out most light sources, try an eye mask, which will stop most light from hitting your retinas through the thin skin of your eyelids. When visiting the bathroom at night, try to make sure that the lights are kept low. Light hitting the retina is what's known as a "circadian alerting signal," and this can prevent the secretion of melatonin and disrupt your sleep.

Body temperature experiences a significant decline at nighttime, signaling to our brain that it's time to sleep. This decreased heat production and increased heat loss before bedtime flips on your brain and body's "time-for-bed" switches and helps you fall asleep. Research shows that keeping your room temperature between 65 and 72 degrees Fahrenheit is optimal when it comes to sleep hygiene.[46]

Noise can easily disrupt sleep for many people, especially if you've ever raised young children. If you're easily woken up by noise, earplugs are a great idea to prevent sleep disruption.

Avoid Caffeine Past 3 p.m.

Avoid any caffeine 4-6 hours before bedtime. This sounds like obvious advice, but a walk past the Starbucks in our neighborhood at 7 p.m. indicates that people are really not taking the advice seriously. Caffeine blocks the adenosine receptor. Adenosine is responsible for making us feel sleepy. Adenosine is supposed to build throughout the day and it plays a key role in sleep homeostasis, i.e., the body's natural way to make you feel sleepy in order to maintain adequate sleep. Caffeine interferes with this process. Many of us will reach for a cup of coffee during the circadian dip in the mid-afternoon, and this should be the last one of the day.

Eat Melatonin-Rich Foods.

Melatonin is the hormone which regulates sleep. It is produced in the brain. Crucially, it can cross the blood brain barrier (BBB) from the gut. This means that we can eat foods rich in melatonin to boost sleep quality.

Research suggests that melatonin-rich tart cherries (and cherry juice) in particular can increase sleep time, decrease the amount of time it takes to fall asleep, and also the number of times you wake up during the night.[47] Take note that dried cherries don't count.

Tart cherry juice is not available in all countries and it can be expensive, so alternative foods high in melatonin include: tomatoes, walnuts, almonds, goji berries, mustard seeds, and fenugreek.

The pineal gland is responsible for the synthesis of melatonin as a response to darkness and part of the circadian rhythm which we will look at shortly.[48] Keeping your circadian rhythm in sync with your current time zone is beneficial for vitality and energy which is why jetlag can make you feel so sleepy.

So should you supplement melotonin? Whilst supplements have their place, eating foods rich in the nutrient is more beneficial as they often contain other helpful compounds and phytochemicals that aid with the full absorption and synthesis of the nutrient into the body.

It is important to consider that melatonin production decreases with advancing age, leading to insomnia and changes to our circadian rhythm. Eat melatonin rich foods from the list mentioned can be a great hack to avoid this.

Listen to Binaural Beats.

The idea behind this hack is that by playing sounds of different frequencies into each ear, specific brain waves can be induced, including delta (sleep), theta (relaxation), beta (concentration), and so on. In the left ear, a sound oscillating at a specific frequency is played while a corresponding sound, played a slightly different frequency, is played into the right ear. The difference between both sounds might seem small, being between 2 and 30 hertz (Hz). Nonetheless, the brain, being an electro-chemical machine, generates its own waves as a bi-product of its neurons firing and signaling each other.

Each one of these waves is very finely-tuned and can be picked up on an electroencephalograph (EEG) as a "brain wave."

During sleep, the brain generates waves from its activities which resonate at about 1-3Hz. For readers who listen to music – a bass sound resonates at around 40Hz. When we are awake, the frequency is much higher and the brain can emit many different types of waves from different regions. Research shows that binaural beats can actually influence our brain waves.[49] See next page for a complete list of brain waves and their frequencies.

Hacking binaural beats requires wearing headphones or earphones, so this isn't necessarily practical for sleeping. Although we don't recommend trying to hack your sleep with binaural beats while you're actually sleeping, playing the sounds for 15 minutes *before* sleeping appears to be a promising area for more research.

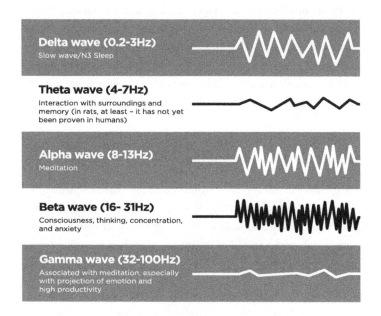

Delta wave (0.2-3Hz)
Slow wave/N3 Sleep

Theta wave (4-7Hz)
Interaction with surroundings and memory (in rats, at least – it has not yet been proven in humans)

Alpha wave (8-13Hz)
Meditation

Beta wave (16- 31Hz)
Consciousness, thinking, concentration, and anxiety

Gamma wave (32-100Hz)
Associated with meditation, especially with projection of emotion and high productivity

Meditate Before Sleep.

Studies have found that meditating before sleep increases the quality of sleep and reduces the feeling of fatigue after a lack of sleep.[50] Research shows that experienced meditators enjoy higher proportions of the essential N3 sleep phase, which is key to energy replenishment, repair, and brain cleaning. This may work though increasing melatonin secretion, which, as we have seen, is crucial for sleep. Secretion of melatonin in turn increases vasodilation, the mechanism which allows toxins to be removed from the brain.

You don't need to be a lifelong meditator to get the benefits of meditating. A Harvard study of a group of non-meditators who, over a period of just 8 weeks, meditated for an average of just 27 minutes per day, showed changes to the brain in the regions related to empathy, emotional regulation, and thinking.[51] One of the huge benefits of mindful meditation for sleep is that, with practice, it can be done without headphones or sleep aids just before sleeping. This makes for a practical hack with many other benefits for energy and vitality. In the final section of this book you will learn more about mindful meditation and the different types, as well as some mindful meditation exercises such as the bodyscan meditation.

Bio Hack 5 | Circadian Rhythm

Even as babies in our mother's womb we already have a schedule, a sense of night and day. Since before we are born, our body is already regulating our sleep and wake patterns, yet it is more sophisticated than we might imagine and of the most importance when it comes to energy and vitality.

The internal clock is so fundamental to our existence, that all organisms synchronize their physiology, behavior and metabolism to the 24-hour solar cycle. Living beings from plants and insects to mammals optimize their health according to external signs that allow them to anticipate responses in accordance to environmental changes. This internal clock is called our circadian rhythm.

The circadian rhythm is defined by four unique characteristics.

1) First, the circadian rhythm mimics the 24-hour solar cycle. It takes both light and darkness to tune our internal clock and the word "circadian" is derived from the Latin for "Almost a day."

2) The second characteristic of this cycle is that even in the absence of external signs such as sunlight, the periodic pattern is maintained. This is due to it having an internal regulation and maintenance system.

3) Thirdly, although our circadian rhythm is mainly guided by internal factors, it is able to adjust to external signs, such as light.

4) Finally, in humans, the most prominent circadian rhythm is the sleep/wake cycle.

Over millions of years, living organisms have run according to these biological rhythms. These circadian rhythms are present in all animals, even bacteria. The rhythms modulate many important physiological functions including body temperature, hormone secretions, and – crucially for energy – the sleep/wake cycle.

Most humans experience peak alertness and attention at 10 a.m. For most, our energy dips to a minimum at around 3 pm and this is because our body reflects the regular patterns of external temperature where the temperature usually peaks in the afternoon. These two peaks and troughs are true for most, however there are early risers and late settlers. Although this alertness pattern is most common in humans, it is not an exact science for all. For 10% of the population their peak alertness occurs significantly earlier and for 20% of the population, their lowest attention point occurs significantly later on in the evening. It is estimated that what defines us as early risers or night owls is 47% inherited. For this reason, early risers and night owls may never be able to fully adapt or change their predisposition. Once an early bird, always an early bird.

Although the master clock for the sleep/wake cycle is in an area of the brain called the hypothalamus, each cell of our body has its own rhythm that oscillates in a semi-independent manner. When our body and our circadian rhythms are in tune, there are important functions that oscillate at par. For example, when sleeping, the melatonin and vasopressin hormones are secreted, the brain waves grow in length and therefore slow down, and the glucose concentration is at its peak. All these systems are independent, but in states of good health, they tend to work in a synchronized way despite the independence. This genetic bias of these rhythms is a major factor, so profound in fact, that the circadian rhythms of human cells in vitro i.e. in a petri dish correlate with the rhythms of the person they were taken from.

In extraordinary situations, when you're lucky enough to travel through time zones and unlucky enough to get jet lag or when working in the night shifts, these systems lose their synchronization. When the natural sleep/wake patterns are disrupted, they tend to lead to high glucose tolerance and low insulin when eating. It also leads to low levels of hormones that control appetite, called ghrelin and leptin, which means feeling hungrier. It is for this reason that there is a strong correlation between the desynchronization of your sleep/wake rhythm and being overweight.

Unfortunately with age, it becomes harder for us to reconcile the interruptions to our day/night routines. It is harder for us to adapt to new time zones or adjust to non-traditional work schedules, such as working late or early in the morning.

Age also affects our hormone levels. During high-school and college years, hormonal changes lead humans to increase socialization prompting adolescents to begin staying up late. This lack of sleep usually affects how alert teenagers are throughout the day and why getting up seems like such a monumental challenge for teenagers. Most teenagers identify themselves as night owls, but only 7% of teenagers will continue being night owls in adulthood.

Age is not the only factor that plays a role in our sleep hygiene i.e. how well we sleep. Our sex hormones are also a major factor. It is known that women experience more challenges than men at maintaining good sleep hygiene. This difference usually becomes more noticeable over the years and this is due to both physiological and social reasons. While there has been a shift from traditional social roles in a family regarding women, statistically women still play the leading role in parental responsibilities at nighttime. The hormonal fluctuations during the monthly cycle of a woman entail changes in progesterone and estrogen levels. The level of these hormones in our body influence how fast we fall asleep, how many times we wake up at night time and how fast we reconcile sleep. Menopause and pre-menopause manifest their own hormonal changes and therefore present their own sleep challenges and disruptions to our circadian rhythms, meaning less energy and vitality and more fatigue.

While our brain is the main regulator of our sleep/wake cycle, biological clocks can be seen in virtually all tissues and organisms, from flies to humans. The circadian rhythm is so biologically rooted within us that it is able to adjust even in blindness. It is not necessary to have fully functioning eyes to adjust the circadian clock. This is because humans have non-visual photo-receptor cells. The most powerful environmental synchronizer is the light / dark cycle. Think about it: the light bulb, invented in 1879, is a recent addition to humanity, which is currently clocking 200,000 years of evolution. The only light bulb that's been around during the entire evolution of our species is the sun. Life on earth is very much tuned to this ultimate source of vitality. It's even been worshiped as a deity for millennia, and for good reason.

However, our rhythms can be disrupted, especially by light (or the absence of it) and the dysregulation of circadian rhythm is associated with many disorders, including metabolic disease and neuropsychiatric disorders including bipolar disorder,[52] anxiety,[53] depression,[54] schizophrenia,[55] and sleep disorders.[56]

The circadian rhythm is a survival system which synchronizes our internal ability to adjust to environmental factors. It not only controls when we feel sleepy and hungry, but also a long list of other internal processes, including the daily regulation of body temperature, neurotransmitter levels, sympathetic activation (your fight, flight and freeze mechanism), energy metabolism (e.g., lipolysis, gluconeogenesis, insulin sensitivity, basal metabolic rate). All very complex but suffice to say that these are all important areas linked to our energy levels and feelings of vitality. The circadian rhythm is, without a doubt, an important are of focus.[57]

Although cells can have their own circadian rhythm, the "master clock" is in an area of the hypothalamus called the suprachiasmatic nuclei (SNC). This particular area is responsible for autonomic actions such as our breathing and heart rate.[58]

Although there is a master clock in the SNC, each cell seems to have its own rhythm. When the system is in sync, important functions oscillate together. For example, when we sleep, the hormones melatonin and vasopressin are secreted, brain waves slow down, and glucose concentration is at its highest, all of which are separately oscillating independent systems that are not linked or inter-dependent. The cells of each system are synchronized to their individual circadian rhythms. Think about it like an orchestra, with the SNC as the conductor. When all of the instruments are in sync, we have a harmonious symphony, when they are not, we have a proverbial train wreck.

The circadian rhythms are adapted to the environmental factors that act as synchronizers or what's known in biology as zeitgebers. Think of them as cues that our body takes from the environment. Although light/darkness is the most important cue, we should not underestimate the power of our meal schedule and our behaviors. These are so relevant that the best way to overcome jet lag is to adjust immediately to the meal schedule of the new time zone. This also has an impact on your levels of fatigue in your home time zone too, so try to stick with a regular meal schedule as closely as possible to avoid confusing your circadian rhythms.

Certain other behaviors are capable of acting as zeitgebers or cues too. Watching television before going to sleep suppresses the production of melatonin, which is the hormone that helps us sleep and maintain the sleep cycle. As you'd expect, the time you sleep, and when you sleep, has an impact on your circadian clock. Not enough sleep decreases the production of rhythmic genes in our organs. So much so that the cycle of transcription of blood cells is slowed i.e. we make less blood cells.

Although the circadian rhythm does not depend entirely on external factors, it is highly influenced by long-term exposure to light and darkness. Many people who work night shifts suffer from insomnia when they sleep during the day. One way to avoid this is to avoid sun exposure early in the morning. You can do this by wearing dark glasses after finishing the shift, getting to a darkened house or apartment as soon as possible and waking up when there is still light outside. Starting the day with direct sunlight and doing daily exercise will help to make the desynchronization less noticeable. It is important to know that most accidents caused by human error usually happen at night, from the fatigue of pilots resulting in the deaths of hundreds of passengers, to catastrophic events such as Chernobyl. Trying to force the body to adjust to being awake at night can be a recipe for disaster. While night shifts are inevitable for many, the most beneficial thing for your attention, vitality and health is to keep them to a minimum when possible.

Research with sleep deprived volunteers found them to have poor glucose tolerance and lower insulin sensitivity to eating breakfast, neither of which are optimal for your health.

Research studies have shown that the circadian rhythm of some cells is intrinsically linked with energy metabolism in cells through a protein called PGC-1A. As you may recall, this is the coactivator that actives mitochondrial biogenesis.[59] Studies have shown that mice without the PGC-1A gene had disturbed circadian rhythms so the two are closely linked. As we have seen previously, PGC-1A is a key to both energy metabolism and mitochondrial biogenesis, growing more of the power generating engines in each of the body's cells.

The link between PGC-1A may explain the relationship between what's known as metabolic syndrome and a disturbed circadian rhythm. Metabolic syndrome is a combination of diabetes, high-blood pressure and obesity. Changes to sleep patterns and a disturbed circadian rhythm could be affecting how our bodies use energy at the cellular level. There are many influences on the circadian rhythm as we have seen, the most important of which is light followed by sleep and following a regular meal schedule.

So the science is very interesting and compelling, and you now understand what it takes to maintain a healthy circadian rhythm. How else can you take advantage of your circadian rhythm to enjoy more energy, vitality and less fatigue?

By simply knowing which times of day you're likely to have more energy or to be more wakeful, you can schedule high-priority tasks for the most optimal times. Tasks that involve complex thought and cognition should be done first. There is more evidence in neuroscience to support putting your toughest tasks first, as we will see later in this book. Psychology research also supports this habit, as well as the theory that willpower runs out throughout the day and therefore is strongest in the morning.

Energy levels are very unique to each individual. There are many factors within each of the 4 Energy Quadrants (biological, neurological, motivational, environmental), and everybody's mix of what works and what doesn't will be very personal. Nonetheless, working early mornings seem to be a factor shared by many successful people through history. Having an early start allows us to get things done before distractions and obligations start piling up. It also allows you to set the tone for the rest of the day, giving you an added sense of control in your life. Scientists have also found that even if you are a night owl, willpower is highest in the morning, which is essential for optimal decision-making. This is one of the reasons why it is easier to follow your diet in the mornings but your decisions might get harder and unhealthier as the day goes by and your energy levels start to diminish.

Our eating schedules affect our body's digestive system and its schedule. This impact explains why night owls are found to have significantly more health problems. They have twice the risk of suffering psychological disorders, a third higher risk of developing diabetes and almost a quarter higher chance to have respiratory disease, neurological problems and gastrointestinal disorders. Apart from objective health, early risers also tend to subjectively score higher in feeling healthier, more alert and score their quality of sleep as higher than night owls.

There is a natural tendency to sleep at certain times which is separate to the circadian rhythm. This natural tendency to sleep is called homeostatic sleep drive. Remember that homeostasis is the body's ability to get its systems back to a steady regular baseline. The circadian rhythm signals us to be more alert at specific times – this is known as the "circadian alerting signal," which we've mentioned previously. The circadian dip, on the other hand, is the period in mid-afternoon where energy levels drop and we feel sleepier. Sleep homeostasis, the circadian alert, and the circadian dip should ideally sync together. Simple morning routines like getting 15-30 minutes of sunlight after waking up can sync circadian rhythm and enhance cognitive and physical function.

So, in conclusion, the circadian rhythm is a very important and complex series of biological systems that operate entirely independently. For our health, wellbeing, and vitality they synchronize with each other and with the light/dark cycle of the day. Your goal is to make sure that your rhythms are working in harmony by sleeping and eating at regular times, getting 15-30 minutes of sunlight each morning on waking, ideally at sunrise. Taking a short 20 minute nap in mid afternoon and prioritizing your most complex tasks for earlier in the day will also help you to ride your circadian rhythm.

Bio Hack 6 | Diet Hacks

Most people want a quick hit, an easy and effective way to boost energy that is neatly pre-packaged and available at their local shops. We scrutinize our research sources very seriously and, when commercial interests could be involved, we take a much closer look on behalf of the consumer.

The foods that we eat have a massive effect on our levels of energy, vitality and fatigue, but it's hard to know what to choose with so much information and so many claims being made. You already know that you should eat a low-fat, high-protein, low-glycemic index (GI) diet rich in leafy green vegetables. You already know that you should eliminate all trans fats (the processed fats typically found in cookies, ice cream and processed foods) and keep the saturated fats to a minimum. Suffice to say, the healthy diet we just described is a prerequisite for feeling higher vitality and energy, but do you know why and what else you can do?

Reduce Processed Fats and Sugar

Processed fats are bad for your brain. We all know that trans fats and saturated fats can increase your risk of heart disease. Even more alarming, a landmark project in the U.S. showed that a diet high in trans and saturated fat is associated with cognitive decline. It's not the first study of its kind to reach this conclusion, but this study was unprecedented because it had an extended timeline, lasting for 6 years.[60] Especially notable was the finding that it isn't the total amount of fat consumed that was associated with cognitive decline; it was the specific *types* of fats. (Other studies warn simply about total fat intake.[61]) Either way, a high-fat diet, especially one that contains saturated and trans fats, is bad for your brain health and energy levels.

Our bodies do need fats, and luckily not all fats are created equal. Monounsaturated fats that are found in nuts, avocados, and olive oil were associated with cognitive improvements when they make up high percentages of fat intake.

A large study showed that a diet high in trans fats is associated not only with lower cognitive performance but also with lower brain volume. It was also found that a diet high in omega-3 and vitamins D, C, and E is associated with higher brain volume and better cognitive performance. We'll come back to omega-3s a little later on. For trans fats, it gets worse, as one of the specific impacts of trans fats is on working memory.[62] Different to your long term memory, working memory is a series of systems connected in the brain that help you to operate consciously throughout the day. It helps you to process your environment, to make decisions and form behaviors based on the new information. As you can imagine, if you're feeling a little foggy or fatigued, you're working memory will be involved in some way.

One particular study, that looked into 1,000 young adult men, showed conclusively that trans fats were associated with poor word recall. It is more evidence that trans fats affect not only cardiovascular health but also brain health and cognition. As we know, cognition is only a part of feeling energized, our mood also contributes significantly to our feelings of vitality. Unfortunately, trans fats have also been linked to depression, showing that it can negatively affect your subjective feelings of energy and vitality.[63]

Trans fats and saturated fats are not the only foods to avoid for the sake of energy and vitality. The effect of a high-sugar diet on mental functioning is very worrying too. In fact, research points to a high-fat and high-sugar diet capable of altering the hippocampus and maintaining a vicious cycle in which decision making is significantly impaired.[64] High-fat/high-sugar diets have been linked to brain inflammation and Brain Derived Neurotrophic Factor (BDNF) repression in the hippocampus.[65] This affects memory and nerve development. We will come back to BDNF later in the book.

The energy hack to be learned here is to keep your energy intake from healthy sources. Protein should make up the bulk of your diet, supplemented by some mono and polyunsaturated fats from fish, olive oil, avocados, and nuts as well as some carbohydrates from low-glycemic sources, specifically whole grains and vegetables.

As with fats, not all sugars are equal. Fructose comes in two forms, depending on the source. Fructose is the sugar found in fruit, but there is also a less healthy version in the corn sugar found in many sweetened foods. We already know that the liver can only process a small amount of fructose at a time. Studies show that a high-sugar diet that includes corn sugar is associated with cognitive decline on a wide range of tests. On the other hand, fructose from natural fruit sources had no negative effect whatsoever on cognition.[66] Sucrose, otherwise known as table sugar, is not much better, with tests confirming the same result. This is not surprising, as sucrose is 50% fructose to begin with.

Processed fructose appears to be linked not only to inflammation, as we mentioned earlier, but also to the metabolism of glucose. The effect seem to relate to insulin resistance facilitated by fructose and its interaction with triglyceride levels. Increased triglycerides from fats increases insulin resistance, which in turn affects glucose utilization. Insulin resistance is when the cells of your body simply stop absorbing glucose, even though insulin is signaling to do so. Your body will be full of glucose that's floating around in circulation, but it can't use it. Think of it as a car with a tank full of gas that can't make it into the engine. The worrying factor here is that triglycerides can cross the BBB and can, therefore, decrease the ability of your brain to use the glucose that it needs to function.

Although we need insulin in small amounts for memory and cognitive functioning, insulin is not harmful, insulin resistance and Type 2 diabetes is.[67] A body that's regularly swamped with large amounts of insulin can become insulin resistant through Type 2 diabetes. Insulin resistance is a cause of this type of diabetes, in which the cells simply stop absorbing glucose from the blood altogether even when insulin tells it to. Glucose, as we know, is critically important for brain function, so insulin resistance can lead to declining mental functioning, due to neurons not absorbing glucose properly. Eating a high-Glycemic Index (GI) carbohydrate and high-fat diet leads to Type 2 diabetes which, for energy hackers and anyone feeling fatigue, should be avoided at all costs.

High-GI carbohydrates are carbs such as sucrose, processed fructose i.e. corn sugar, potatoes, and white bread, all of which increase insulin levels disproportionately compared to low-glycemic carbs such as broccoli, soy, and whole grains.

Canadian Paralympic athlete Eliza Linnéa Gatzwiller confided details of her diet to us in an interview. She is a remarkable athlete who has competed at a top level despite suffering two brain tumors, five strokes, and five heart attacks in her life. At 40, she is one of the oldest competing Paralympic swimmers in Canada. She trains in the pool every day starting at 5:30 a.m. and is a winner through and through. Early on in her recovery Eliza worked with a nutritionist and friend who changed the way she has eaten to this day. Eliza takes no supplements and gets all of her nutrition from natural sources, but she is clear that her energy comes from eating a low-GI diet which consists of pasta as the main source of carbohydrate. Her goal is to avoid the crashes, she mentioned, referring to the feeling of fatigue that we experience when our energy levels peak and then plummet after eating high-GI foods.

We strongly recommend following Eliz'a example, and to get your carbs from low GI sources too. Getting your fats from fish, avocados, nuts and occasionally a little olive oil is also important as you've learned. Most importantly, you should avoid fast sugars, trans fats and highly saturated fats as a baseline habit for avoiding fatigue and feeling more energy and vitality. It won't be easy, but you can try for just one meal per day or even week. As you get more comfortable and familiar, you can scale to replacing more meals per week with healthy meals. You can finally make it part of your day, with the goal of all meals being healthy meals. Start today!

Reduce Alcohol

You're a busy person, so we won't waste your time telling you about the long-term effects of alcohol on your health. You already know the effects of liver cirrhosis, diabetes, and Wernicke-Korsakoff Syndrome (OK, maybe not that one). As you might have experienced, after 2-3 hours of alcohol consumption, our energy is impaired. Most heavy long-term drinkers will experience cognitive decline in the form of a shrinking brain and a decreased ability for abstract thinking. Even visuospatial abilities, like remembering where you put the car keys, can be affected. Heavy alcohol consumption causes brain damage, and the effects are the same for long-term social drinkers who drink more than 21 drinks per week. Even light to moderate drinkers who have been drinking for over 10 years have been revealed in studies to have the same level of cognitive decline as a detoxified alcoholic.

The Center of Disease Control describes alcohol as affecting "every organ in the body. It is a central nervous system depressant that is rapidly absorbed from the stomach and small intestine into the bloodstream." Read it: alcohol is a depressant. That's right, and for those of you looking for higher energy and vitality, alcohol is clearly not optimal. As we mentioned earlier in the book, try to limit your drinking to no more than 2 drinks per session, no more than twice per week.

Beetroot

The food choices we make are extremely important and are not only limited to what we should avoid. There are a large number of foods which are beneficial to energy and vitality, and we have listed them in this book. We have chosen foods which have been proven to be beneficial for cognition and to enhance energy. Our aim is to help you make the right choices.

Among the various nutritious benefits of beetroot is vasodilation. As we mentioned earlier, vasodilation is a very important process for increasing the amount of blood supplied to the brain. Beetroot's effects on vasodilation are due to its high nitric oxide content. The endothelium that lines our arteries, dilates in the presence of nitric oxide. This means that the artery expands and more blood can flow through it.

A review of beetroot juice supplementation in athletes showed that beetroot juice can improve cardiorespiratory endurance, specifically by increasing efficiency. This means that less oxygen is required by muscles, which, as we know, is a good thing, considering the damaging effects of too much oxygen on the body. In both the muscles and brain, the utilization of nitric oxide appears to act on the area of energy expenditure.[68]

In a small pilot study into the effects of beetroot juice on cerebral blood flow, beetroot juice was found to lower cerebrovascular resistance and benefiting circulation in the brain. This is due to vasodilation allowing the brain tissue to absorb significantly more nutrients.[69] This is highly favorable for energy and vitality.

Beetroot is an exciting nutritional supplement worthy of more research, but don't start gulping jugs of beetroot juice just yet. Consuming two rations of beets per week, ideally prior to exercise, would be an effective hack. A good philosophy is to think of helping the body and not forcing it. Like anything that's forced, there's a chance it could break. It must be noted that beetroot juice lowers blood pressure, so those with low blood pressure should refrain from this particular hack.

Purple Grape Juice

Interest in red grapes has increased since the observation of the so-called "French paradox." This paradox is founded in the observation that people living in the Mediterranean have a lower probability of cardiovascular problems, despite a diet high in fats. Red wine, specifically the flavonoids in wine, have been considered to be of great relevance to this effect. Flavonoids are compounds common in nature and in the plant kingdom. They help to determine the color of flowers and give plants UV protection. In humans, grape juice has a range of health benefits and has been shown to be cardio-protective, antioxidant, anti-inflammatory, anti-cancer, and antimicrobial. This is, however, a book about energy, vitality, and combating fatigue, so how can it help with our goal?

Researchers from United Kingdom revealed that "purple grape juice can acutely enhance aspects of cognition and mood." Although the researchers could only hypothesize as to the reasons for the positive effects, they pointed towards improved cerebral blood flow and glucose utilization as possibilities.[70]

Researchers believe that most of the health benefits of grape juice could be ascribed to one specific flavonoid called anthocyanin.[71] Anthocyanin is a potent antioxidant, however, researchers are still unclear on the effect of anthocyanins on cognition and mood. One of anthocyanin's benefits to the brain is the prevention of neurodegenerative processes by inhibiting neuro-inflammation and by reducing oxidative stress.

Beware that many fruit juices are composed of artificial flavors or low percentages of concentrate. Also, almost always, juices come with added sugar. In liquid form, sugar can spike insulin and is counterproductive for higher energy and vitality. The best option to get your red grape benefits is to eat the grapes or to drink pure, sugar-free grape juice.

Ginseng

We know that many readers will pick up information from the internet and may be using, or curious to use, specific foods or supplements to fight fatigue and feel more energized. In this, and other sections, we have take a close look at the supporting evidence for many of the most popular so that you can make a balanced choice.

Although ginseng is currently very popular, there is little evidence that ginseng has a real long-term benefit on energy and vitality in healthy humans. There is, nonetheless, promising evidence that ginseng can have beneficial effects in another useful area.

In a review by scientists at the University of Florida's School of Medicine, ginseng was found to have an effect on neurodegenerative illnesses due to its anti-inflammatory, anti-oxidative and anti-apoptosis properties. They stressed, however, that nearly all studies were on rats and mice. They also pointed out that the effects of ginseng appeared neuroprotective (as opposed to enhancing) and claimed that it could protect the brain from damage by maintaining a state of optimal functioning. The results are promising because the ginseng, as we know, has neuroprotective qualities. It's worth remembering, however, that many neurologically-focused therapies and treatments improve the cognitively impaired but have little or no effect on healthy individuals.

On balance, if you are already using ginseng and getting good results, then by all means, continue to use it. If you're evaluating whether it should be part of your diet, our suggestion is to try it in its natural root form 1st. The high price of the supplement is quite prohibitive and the direct link to fatigue and vitality is so far inconclusive.

L-Carnitine

L-carnitine is an amino acid that is processed in the liver and kidneys, with vitamin C being an essential component in that process. The sources highest in L-carnitine are milk and red meat, but it's also found in nuts and legumes.

If you're well rested and in good shape, L-carnitine may not give you the A-game cognitive boost you're looking for. A review by researchers of the available studies drew the conclusion that there was, as of 2017, no credible evidence to support L-carnitine's credentials in improving cognition in healthy people.[72]

Many studies into the effects of L-carnitine have focused on the cognitively impaired. They found promising results, specifically patients with dementia and older adults. A large high-quality trial is required to prove any benefits for L-carnitine for cognitive performance in healthy adults, however. Some researchers have suggested that there may be benefits for sleep-deprived or stressed healthy adults but, alas, there's just no proof yet to back this up.

The reason that researchers hypothesize that sleep-deprived and stressed adults may benefit from it is because L-carnitine is not required for the production of ATP energy in the brain. It is speculated that when we are stressed or fatigued, our production of ATP may be compromised. L-carnitine could offer support and alleviate the symptoms of fatigue by assisting in the oxidation of fats (although, of course, sleep will always be the best option).[73]

Creatine

Creatine is found in red meat and fish, and is often consumed by athletes as a supplement in powdered form called creatine monohydrate. Creatine is converted to creatinine by the liver and kidneys, and it's stored in the muscles as phosphocreatine. Phosphocreatine is a high-energy backup for cells and can regenerate ATP when the cells need it.

Remember, the brain cannot store energy, but it too uses phosphocreatine. At times of intense brain activity, phosphocreatine drops very quickly as it works to backs up the ATP.

For mental energy and vitality, creatine shows real promise as a neuroprotective supplement.[74] Trials in rats and mice have shown that creatine can enhance mitochondrial function whilst decreasing the evil oxygen reactive species (ROS) that can cause damage to cells.[75] That means it enhances the power plant while limiting the toxic and cell-destroying effects which would normally be a byproduct of producing more energy than usual.

In humans, there is credible evidence that creatine offers a cognitive boost relating to mood, and also to executive functions such as reasoning and logic (especially when sleep deprived). This effect is due to the fact that sleep deprivation reduces the amount of creatine in the brain. So, consuming creatine-rich foods or a supplement which soon crosses the blood brain barrier (BBB) is an effective way of restoring the creatine drop in the brain.

It should be noted though that all of the human subjects in the studies into fatigue, sleep deprivation, and creatine had already undergone a loading phase of at least seven days. That means the test subjects had taken a larger dose for seven days to build up their bodies' stores of creatine.[76,77] We therefore recommend that you too start with a short loading phase which is often recommended when taking creatine supplementation for the 1st time. Remember to closely follow the manufacturer's recommendations when taking any supplement. The loading phase should be stopped after a few days and the dose reduced to the recommended level.

L-Tyrosine

Tyrosine shows promise for performance in high-stress situations. This is because tyrosine can enhance the synthesis and release of both dopamine and norepinephrine. Norepinephrine is the brain version of the hormone adrenaline. Dopamine and norepinephrine are both key players in the stress response in the brain. At times of stress, our norepinephrine/adrenaline system is activated, and the norepinephrine neurotransmitter is turned over and quickly depleted. The depletion of norepinephrine can leave the person with feelings of helplessness and anxiety.

Tyrosine is very specific in action. Increased circulating tyrosine only acts when there is a deficiency, and there appears to be no benefit to healthy adults who are not stressed. This offers an excellent hack for readers who may be experiencing stress and anxiety. Simply keeping the tyrosine levels high has been noted as safe by researchers, as our bodies frequently have high tyrosine exposure with no side effects: it's only used when needed. Foods high in tyrosine are cheese, beef, chicken, soybeans, fish, nuts, eggs, dairy, and whole grains.

Another interesting fact is that tyrosine is a precursor of natural antidepressants. For that reason, and because it can protect the brain from stress, eating foods with a high tyrosine content is a great way to balance your mood."

L-Histidine

L-histidine is one of the least abundant amino acids. It is the precursor to histamine, a neurotransmitter which controls our sense of wakefulness (we will discuss histamine more thoroughly in the next chapter). Increasing levels of L-histidine increases the amount of histamine in the brain, making it a possible energy hack.

It is likely that increasing levels of L-histidine doesn't necessarily increase neuronal firing of histamine receptors.

L-histidine is converted in the brain to the neurotransmitter histamine. One study in Japan found that a low-L-histidine diet can lead to neurological symptoms, including anxiety.[78] This suggests that the brain needs dietary L-histidine to function optimally and that histamine has a positive effect on other neurotransmitters, such as serotonin. Eating food high in L-histidine is therefore important for our more subjective feelings of vitality and energy.

Foods which are high in L-histidine but low in dietary histamine (which we don't want), such as beef and soy beans, are essential for alertness and mental energy as well as maintenance of a healthy immune system and gut. Remember to be wary of ingesting dietary histamine. Dietary histamine is histamine which has already been converted from the amino acid L-histidine on or in the food. *Fermented* soy products, processed meats, beer, and red wine will reduce your levels of L-histidine by interfering with absorption in the stomach. We only want our L-histidine turning into histamine after it crosses the blood brain barrier and not before.

Since research shows that a low-L-histidine diet affects the amounts of histamine in the brain, ingesting adequate amounts is a must. There is a direct correlation: ingesting more varied sources of high-quality protein, especially vegetable sources (and not only red meat and poultry), is a good way to boost your protein intake without affecting heart health as well as boosting your feelings of vitality.

Iodine

Iodine is taken up by plants from the soil. If the local soil contains little iodine, neither does the plant. Unfortunately, 32 countries, including the UK and Australia, have iodine-deficient soil. Many of us are used to receiving extra supplementation of iodine from iodized salt. However, most of us now eat less salt, and the salt industry no longer adds iodine to its salt in all countries. But is iodine important for energy, and how so?

A lack of iodine can lead to a range of health problems so numerous and common that they are labeled the "iodine deficiency disorders." When it comes to energy, iodine deficiency can result in impaired mental function.

Iodine is stored in the thyroid gland, and a lack of iodine can result in goiter. A goiter is a large lump that can grow on the side of the neck as a result of the thyroid gland swelling up to get more iodine. The thyroid produces hormones that are vital for energy metabolism and homeostasis, so a functioning thyroid gland is critically important for energy and vitality.

Iodine consumption is an energy hack, not only because it acts directly on energy metabolism, but also because we are highly likely to be deficient in it. So, how to hack it?

Seawater contains iodine and there are high concentrations in shellfish and seaweed. As shellfish can, on occasion, contain harmful toxins and bacteria, seaweed, or "wakame" as it's known in Japan, is a great option for increasing your iodine levels naturally.

Another option is to increase your intake of cereals, fish, and fruit. Research on elite wheelchair basketball players showed that their diet was deficient in iodine as well as other important micronutrients. The players were able to increase their levels of the essential micronutrients by eating a diet high in cereal, fish and fruits.

Increasing levels of iodine naturally through eating the right foods is preferable to a supplement in tablet form, although supplementation could be an interim solution.[79] The reason for naturally increasing through food intake is that: a) food has a much wider profile of micronutrients and phytochemicals, and b) too much iodine is as harmful as too little.

Iron

When we think of iron, we often think of the breakfast cereals that are "fortified" with iron. The very fact that our breakfast cereal needs to be fortified, says a lot about the intrinsic nutritional profile of the basic ingredients. We may, however benefit, from the fortification. The Center for Disease Control labels iron as the most common nutritional deficiency worldwide.

Iron is a key component in energy metabolism hormones. It is also a component of hemoglobin and myoglobin, which transport oxygen throughout the body. As you can imagine, iron is vital for energy. A severe lack of iron can result in anemia, which include fatigue and low energy.[80] Hence, eating foods high in iron is advised.

Iron deficiency can damage not only energy levels and vitality, but also mental performance. Studies have shown impaired cognitive performance in iron-deficient subjects. It has also been observed that iron deficiency decreases energy metabolism. Studies also found that the magnitude of performance reduction is directly linked to the amount of iron in the bloodstream.[81] This means, the less iron you have, the less able you are to perform mental tasks.

Iron is best absorbed by the consumption of iron-rich foods. The best sources of iron are:

- Red meat, pork, and poultry
- Dark green leafy vegetables, such as spinach
- Lentils and beans

Iron absorption can benefit from the presence of Vitamin C. We usually get enough Vitamin C from our regular diet. Just adding a salad dressing made with lemon juice to salads will also help to raise levels in the bloodstream.

Iron, as with iodine, is an excellent hack for higher energy and vitality. Again, not only are you likely to be deficient in it, but it is also vital for energy, both physical and mental. It's all about the food choices that we make. If we choose whole foods such as the ones mentioned so far, we are far more likely to receive the right nutrient profile for higher energy levels.

Omega-3 Fatty Acids + Vitamins C, D, and E

Consumption of omega-3 fatty acids, typically found in fatty fish such as salmon, is a must for any serious energy hacker. Omega-3 is high in a substance called DHA, the acronym for docosahexaenoic acid, which is a major component of brain cells that allows them to fire effectively and efficiently. Unfortunately, our bodies find it very difficult to synthesize DHA, so we need a sufficient dietary intake to maintain optimal levels.

Omega-3 supplementation has been shown to improve processing speed, executive functioning and recognition recall memory. Omega-3s can also increase plasticity in the hippocampus and the hypothalamus. In fact, omega-3s have the same effect on neuroplasticity and BDNF levels (which we'll come to later) as a good run or gym session. Interestingly, this effect can be even stronger when paired with exercise.

Aside from the boost to neurons, omega-3s also help with vasodilation creating a positive effect on cognition.[82] Omega-3s influence a specific type of vasodilation called "flow-mediated vasodilation." This signifies the extent to which blood vessels can expand under the pressure of the blood flow itself.

Going straight to the sources, omega-3s are found abundantly in salmon, tuna, and avocados. Omega-3s are an essential energy hack: they offer a range of benefits both neuroprotective and cognitively enhancing. Eating the right type of oily fish, such as salmon or tuna, as part of our diet will increase your omega-3 levels and your iodine intake at the same time – two hacks in one!

Science advocates for a diet high in omega-3s as well as in vitamins C, D, and E to achieve a better cognitive performance. Vitamins C, D, and E are found in foods such as dark leafy greens, pineapple, mango, oranges, and yellow bell peppers (for vitamin C); fatty fish such as tuna (for vitamin D); and almonds, spinach, and avocados (for vitamin E).

Omega-3s and vitamins C, D, and E are highly recommended as energy hacks. We suggest you add these to your diet on a daily basis.

Alpha Lipoic Acid (ALA)

It is highly unlikely that you are currently ingesting sufficient quantities of ALAs. This is due to the fact that the main source of ALAs is offal meat – i.e., organ meats such as brain, liver and heart. ALAs, however, have a few powerful effects, for energy in particular.[83]

ALAs reside in cells with a key function on mitochondria energy metabolism. They are considered to be an antioxidant and energy regulator. This is partly due to their ability to recycle other antioxidants, including vitamins C and E. ALAs have also been shown to improve triglyceride levels in liver tissue, which is an indication that fat is being metabolized more effectively. ALAs are readily absorbed into the body and play a key role in glucose metabolism within brain cells. Even more impressively, ALAs contributes to cellular protection.

Considering the difficulty in getting ALA through food sources, as well as the effects on energy metabolism and cellular protection, ALA is a strong candidate for supplementation and a worthy energy hack which we recommend. As usual, remember to follow the dosage recommended by the manufacturer.

Summary

The body is an elegant and complex machine for converting your food into usable energy, analogous to a refining plant which turns oil into gasoline. It's hard not to be amazed by the sophistication of the complex sequence of systems and processes involved in turning the food we eat into the energy we enjoy. It is often said that any system is as strong as its weakest link, this is what's known as the Theory of Constraints. Surely, if we had no teeth to chew with, or if our small intestine was not functioning well, or if we had a problem with insulin sensitivity (like diabetes), or any other affected processes, the functioning of our whole system would be impacted. The hacks in this book give you concrete ways to maximize your biological health to enjoy more energy, vitality and to feel less fatigued, and this starts with your digestive and metabolic systems.

With too little sugar in the bloodstream we become irritable and anxious, which is our body's signal that we need to seek food and restore the balance of glycogen in the body. In emergency situations, like lost in the desert or enduring a fast, where sugar is not available for an extended period, it is possible for the brain to use fat for fuel, in the form of ketones. This is a slow metabolic process for the body which begins with breaking down the fat from either food or lipid fat stores in your body. Your brain and your body, however, are meant to run on glucose derived from carbohydrates or proteins.

Once in the brain, glucose is metabolized and converted to ATP in the mitochondria. Brain cells have hundreds to thousands of mitochondria, representing a very energy-hungry machine that requires a constant supply of glucose from the body. The body, as we have seen, is able to store glucose for times when blood sugar levels are lower. The glycogen, or stored glucose, is then released by the liver signaling the release of fat cells. By that time, you would have hit the next meal. By eating between meals you are calming the neurotransmitters rather than appeasing a pressing sugar need.

Eating low-GI carbs, such as pasta, instead of fast sugars, helps your body to deliver constant streams of energy which, together with a healthy liver and pancreas, will guarantee that the foundations of your energy and vitality are firmly laid.

Safely enhancing your cerebral blood flow through flow-mediated vasodilation, is an energy hack that will help you get more glucose to your brain, where it can be used for mental processes. You can support this with exercise, increasing your intake of omega 3s, beetroot juice and red grapes.

Remember that more oxygen doesn't mean higher cognitive functioning. On the other hand poor air quality will lead to fatigue.

Seven to nine hours of high quality sleep and a minimum of 1.5L of water per day, are fundamentals for energy and vitality. Damaging neurotoxins are only removed during sleep. The blood brain barrier (BBB) becomes more porous when we are sleep deprived. Water, on the other hand, maintains the right volume of blood and cerebralspinal fluid. These benefits ensure that the brain has sufficient glucose, oxygen, and nutrition for maximum energy.

Taking daily vitamins can be a great way to supplement our diet for some people. Nonetheless, the best way to get our nutrients is by eating the whole foods that contain them. Our diet is the main source of our physical energy. It is important to remember *why* we eat and that our body today will be the only body we will have until our last day on Earth. Even though we need certain foods to get optimal levels of energy, the health of our digestive and neural systems also benefit from what we consume.

Remember that calories alone do not equate to more energy. The source of energy is the key, with vegetables and lean meats as the best sources, together with a small quantity of healthy fats from nuts, seeds, avocados and fish. It is much harder for your body to use the energy stored in saturated and trans fats, and they have strong negative effects on feelings of vitality so avoid these as much as possible.

You also learned in this chapter that there are many nutrients that are important for energy and vitality including iodine, iron, omega 3s with vitamins A, C, D and E all from natural food sources. Creatine and ALA can offer benefits through supplementation.

The key to this chapter is to make your choices and to be consistent with your diet and lifestyle changes. Start with a day, grow to a week and then a month. It is the consistency which will deliver the results which we promise you, will be worth the effort.

Take a moment now to imagine what your life could be like if you had more vitality and energy, and less fatigue. From there plan your diet and lifestyle changes based on what you've learned and start your journey today. Good luck.

NEUROLOGICAL ENERGY

Energy in the form of ATP delivers the physical energy supply that we need in order to survive, but it's only part of the story of vitality and that elusive but valuable emotion of feeling truly awake and alive. It's a foundation, but there's more to vitality than just ATP – much, much more.

The feeling of vitality is a subjective experience originating in the brain. We live in a world surrounded by different people, objects, and stimuli of all kinds. These people, objects, and stimuli that surround us are perceived by our brain. Although everything around us has an objective reality, the way we perceive it is subjective. Most of us have seen the picture of the old lady/beautiful woman black and white drawing. Many of us see only the old lady at first, others only the beautiful woman. This same phenomenon applies not only to material realities, but also to emotions and feelings. Reality has to be perceived in order to be processed. The way we perceive things is not only limited to our mechanical neural functions, but is also influenced by our previous experiences, memories, and circumstances. Our perceptions are more complex than what simply impacts our senses. This explains why the same event might trigger different emotions in different people. Likewise, the same amount of biological energy is not perceived the same way by two people despite sharing the same anatomy.

But, how do these perceptions occur? Perceptions occur as interplay of neural connections in specific parts of the beautifully complex brain. Highly sophisticated cellular communication within the brain is more than mere architecture. Neurotransmitters are the proteins that signal specific cells to do specific jobs. Increases in the levels of one neurotransmitter results in increases and decreases in other neurotransmitters. These affect our behavior. Our feelings of stress, vitality, alertness, fatigue, happiness, and joy are under the governance of our neurotransmitters. When we think about vitality – the subjective feeling of being alive, boredom, happiness, and so on – our neurotransmitters are key. Before we take a closer look at each of the neurotransmitters and how they affect our mood, wakefulness, and vitality, it is important to know that mood and vitality are very personal.

Some of us are naturally high-energy people, while others struggle to lift their mood. Neither is better or worse; it just depends on our personality and natural energy baseline. Nonetheless, this means that there is no one-size-fits-all solution when it comes to mood and vitality. All solutions must be adjusted to our personal balance.

Many studies into stimulants, like caffeine and nicotine, point to a productive golden zone of energy and vitality. This magical productive zone can be best described as the middle portion of a U-shaped curve, similar to the one shown opposite.

The bottom axis shows our level of stimulation/stress, and the side axis shows our productivity and vitality levels. Following logic, low stimulation means low productivity and vitality. In other words, stimulation is required to function optimally, both cognitively and physically. An example of this can be observed in the link between impaired cognitive functioning and eating disorders. Specifically, visuospatial reasoning, executive function, decision making, attention allocation, and motor function can be affected in people.

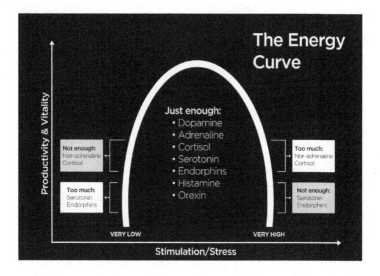

On the other side, too much stress or stimulation inhibits proper cognitive function and physical function, also resulting in low productivity. There are a vast number of studies that show reasoning, executive function, and motor function deficits in people who suffer from clinically diagnosed attention deficiency and hyperactivity.[85][86]

Our objective is to stay at the highest point of the curve. This means achieving a proper level of stimulation is a must to secure optimal performance. It is important to determine our energy baseline. In correlation to our emotional baseline, our energy baseline is susceptible to slow change, depending on our personal circumstances. Our temperament is genetic and neurologically based. It also plays an important role in our energy baseline level, though other factors should be taken into account. As we saw at the beginning of the book, our energy and vitality levels depend on four factors: biological, neurological, motivational, and efficiency. These factors are subjective to variation throughout our lives. Although our temperament determines a certain minimal constant energy baseline, think about your autobiography – think about how you felt when you were a kid waking up in the morning, how you felt waking up after a night out in your early twenties, and how you felt waking up after a night out in your forties. Think about being a first-time parent with sleepless nights, a college student during finals week, or going through an emotionally rough time. It is only normal that our circumstances affect our appetite, sleep pattern, and vitality. The same applies to being in a healthy moment of life, a period of time when you exercise regularly or find yourself in a good emotional stance; a healthy lifestyle will also influence your vitality outcomes.

For those whose energy and mood fall at the bottom end of the arc, both productivity and vitality are low. For those who are bouncing off the walls with energy, productivity is also low, as there is almost always a corresponding lack of clear focus, and anxiety that set in at these levels.

Your job, as an energy hacker, is to determine where you currently are on the U-shaped curve and then, using the hacks in this book, to move yourself into the golden zone of the curve. For example, if your mood, vitality, and energy are low, you may want to address the direct adrenaline, dopamine, and motivation hacks in this book. If you are feeling hyper and at the far end of the curve, you may want to look into serotonin and the efficiency hacks in this book for greater focus. Energy, mood, and vitality are personal to every individual, and it is your responsibility to take ownership in self-appraisal and energy hacking until you are in the golden zone.

As we mentioned before, temperament is genetic and is linked to our neurology.[87] Temperament can be defined as biologically-based characteristic patterns of emotional reactivity and self-regulation that appear early in our childhood.[88] Research has defined the relationship between neuro-cognitive models of temperament and self-regulatory behaviors as effortful control, attention, and executive abilities.[89][90]

Effortful control is the ability to inhibit a dominant emotional response in order to perform a more rational response, detect errors, and engage in planning.

Executive and attention skills underlie effortful control; as these skills develop, we are more able to voluntarily deploy our attention and regulate our emotional and behavioral reactivity, including tendencies such as approach, fear, and anger.[91][92]

This ability to control responses also determines our natural energy levels. Children's natural energy levels are defined by how flexible, active, or cautious they are. These characteristics are constant throughout life and influence our energy baseline enormously.

Most importantly, the biology behind temperament comes down to the production and re-uptake of neurotransmitters. Neurotransmitters are the leading players in energy baseline and in our subjective feeling of energy. Let's take a closer look at these mysterious actors and how they contribute to the grand performance that is our energy.

Histamine

Arguably, when we think about energy and vitality, we think about wakefulness. Histamine, which we introduced in the previous chapter, is, amongst other things, a wakefulness neurotransmitter controlled by a region of the brain called the posterior hypothalamus – your "wakefulness center."

Serotonin, histamine, orexin, dopamine, and adrenaline are vital in our perception of feeling awake. We will look at each of them in detail in this chapter and how to hack each of them without medication or stimulants. One tiny area about the size of a pea, called the tuberomammillary nucleus, releases histamine. Histamine release is highest when we are awake and lowest during sleep. Blocking the breakdown of histamine makes us feel more awake.[93]

Histamine-inducing drugs can be useful to treat sleep problems. Ciproxifan, which targets the H3 histamine receptor of cells, can significantly increase cognitive ability, attention, and wakefulness.[94] The drug is being proposed as a treatment for narcolepsy, a condition in which sufferers can spontaneously fall asleep without warning.[95] It has already been used as a solution for medically diagnosed sleeping problems, but it has not been tested on healthy subjects who are not suffering with sleeping problems so far. It does however demonstrate the importance of histamine for wakefulness, vitality and shaking off that feeling of fatigue.

So we know that histamine works for wakefulness but, outside of pharmacology, there are no hacks to increase the activity of histamine and we wouldn't necessarily want to, the side effects of increasing histamine levels can be intense. Our goal is simply to make sure that our histamine system is functioning optimally. The best way to look after your histamine system is to not expose yourself to allergens for a prolonged period of time. The body has an incredible ability to fight off an allergic reaction for short while, but if exposed for long enough, the system will switch to releasing histamines. Histamines are one of the few neurotransmitters which can increase the permeability of the blood brain barrier (BBB), a situation which should be avoided at all costs.[96] This means that with increased histamine in the bloodstream, sleep can be negatively affected and, as we know, the importance of maintaining grade-A sleep is paramount for fighting fatigue.

One distinction needs to be made between dietary histamine and the amino acid L-histidine which we also briefly explained in the previous chapter. Dietary histamine is L-histidine that has already been converted to histamine on food and is commonly found on fermented foods. L-histidine, an essential amino acid, is found in beef and other protein sources. It is L-histidine that crosses the BBB to be converted to the useful neurotransmitter and it's the *dietary histamine* that can sometimes lead us to an intolerance of it. It's an important distinction for energy, as L-histidine is converted to histamine in the brain, which **is** a process that makes us feel more awake.

Eating adequate protein is a must for maintaining healthy levels of histamine. We must remind ourselves here that the basic building blocks of all neurotransmitters come from amino acids, which pass the BBB and are converted to the neurotransmitters essential for our feelings for vitality and wakefulness. For example, the amino acid L-tryptophan converts to serotonin and from there melatonin; L-tyrosine converts to dopamine, norepinephrine and epinephrine; L-histidine converts to histamine; choline forms acetylcholine; and L-glutamate turns into GABA. These are all essential amino acids which we get form the protein in our diet.

Fermented foods contain *dietary* histamine. These are foods where the L-histidine (the stuff we want) has already been converted to histamine by bacteria in the fermentation process. We only want to consume L-histidine and let our bodies naturally convert it once it's in the brain. Indeed, histamine found on food is often used as a marker of poor food hygiene. Flooding the body with histamine grown on food can lead to a histamine intolerance – but how so?

Research shows histamine intolerance is the result of overexposure and a cumulative effect of histamine buildup in the bloodstream. Histamine levels can be increased in the bloodstream in several ways but the main one is from eating foods that are high in histamine such as fermented foods. This inhibits the action of the compound which breaks down histamine in the bloodstream called Diamine Oxidase which has the ominous acronym, DOA.

The foods that are high in dietary histamine are usually the ones that have undergone fermentation, including cheese, beer, or wine. Citrus fruits too, have the uncanny ability to facilitate the release of histamine from certain cells.[97] Alcohol not only contains histamine but also inhibits the action of DOA. For this reason it is best to avoid it if we aim for a good night's sleep.[98]

Foods that are high in histamine include:

- Fermented alcoholic beverages, especially wine, champagne and beer
- Fermented foods: sauerkraut, vinegar, soy sauce, kefir, kombucha, and natto.
- Vinegar-containing foods: pickles, mayonnaise, olives
- Cured meats: bacon, salami, pepperoni, luncheon meats, and hot dogs

It's worth noting that some detergents, especially water-soluble ones, inhibit DOA in the stomach.[99] For this reason, it is a good idea to make sure your dishes are well rinsed after washing up.

In conclusion, control fermented food intake and consume enough protein in your diet to obtain proper L-histidine levels. This will give your body adequate supply of this neurotransmitter, which is easily depleted and aids absorption amongst other neurotransmitters. As histamine is such an important neurotransmitter for feeling awake, this really is a fundamental hack for anyone feeling fatigued and low on energy.

Orexin

When it comes to wakefulness, orexin is another key neurotransmitter that is intrinsically linked to maintaining constant levels of energy in the body. Orexin appears to increase arousal as a survival mechanism to make us more effective hunters and foragers for food by increasing our alertness.

Keeping orexin levels at optimal, not too high but not too low, is an essential part of balancing your personal U-shaped energy curve and we will share a useful hack with you shortly. Before we do so, the science of orexin is quite fascinating but also complex.

Orexin works in an interplay between serotonin, GABA (which inhibits orexin), noradrenaline (which can do both – but mainly inhibits orexin), and dopamine. Histamine, however, has no effect on orexin. The interplay of orexin with other hormones linked to emotion such as serotonin, adrenaline, and also ghrelin is delightfully complex and not fully understood. As we mentioned, orexin is linked to maintaining constant levels of energy, a process called energy homeostasis, and appears to increase arousal as a survival mechanism. As orexin makes us feel more awake and alert, this appears to make us more effective hunters and foragers for food. Ghrelin is a key here. As we will see, ghrelin is a hormone, mainly produced in the stomach, which signals our need to eat and to wake up in the morning. Increases in ghrelin stimulate more of orexin's wakefulness activity and it can be induced by exercise too. The story goes like this: your stomach becomes empty and shrinks, the shrinking action releases ghrelin and you feel hungry, this then activates orexin which makes you more awake and alert to find food. A pretty neat system!

Glucose and leptin (the hormone that says "stop eating") also puts the brakes on orexin, which makes sense, as orexin is responsible for making us feel alert for the purpose of seeking food.[100] Once we've found food and eaten, orexin has performed one of its vital tasks. Overeating often makes us feel sleepy because leptin suppresses orexin.

So orexin can make us feel sharper but requires us to feel a little hunger. None of us enjoy being hungry, so the question is, how to hack orexin without the hunger pangs?

One possible orexin wakefulness hack is to target oxytocin instead. Orexin is increased by oxytocin.[101] Oxytocin is the hormone that makes us get along with each other, and hacking the oxytocin system is much easier than hacking the orexin system. A good way to get more oxytocin is simply to spend quality time with friends and loved ones.

Emotions have great impact on wakefulness, and the mechanism is complex. The limbic system of the brain, responsible for regulating emotions, can regulate the effects of orexin too. It is hypothesized that orexin neurons receive inputs from the limbic system to trigger a more wakeful state when the need arises. It is suggested that, when we are stressed, the disrupted sleep that often accompanies these stressful periods is due to the emotional limbic system stimulating the greater orexin activity. So, while moderate stress could keep you awake or on the edge of your seat, too much stress is not a good thing and could disrupt your sleep – which is, of course, counterproductive to your energy and vitality. This leads us to the hack to keep orexin in the target zone, self-coaching before bedtime.

Orexin Hack | Self-Coaching Before Bedtime

Self-coaching before bedtime is an excellent way to achieve a good night's sleep as well as higher energy levels the next day. Self-coaching calms the brain. Self-coaching is an activity that heavily involves the thinking part of the brain, the pre-frontal cortex (PFC). The PFC can override the emotional limbic system, and this will reduce orexin's wakefulness activity, which is just what you want before bedtime!

Evidence of this effect comes from former world champion ice skater Owen Edwards, who we interviewed about his winning energy habits. Owen is a driven athlete who still trains today as hard as ever and with a grueling schedule. Owen is a high-energy individual. In our interview Owen cited the need to deal with life issues to stay focused. A natural problem solver, he self-coaches because, as he says, *"I was always trained to analyze things in detail and feel that my brain will not stop until I find a satisfactory answer to any problems I encounter."*

Owen's self-coaching helps to regulate his orexin, dopamine, and serotonin balance, keeping him in the middle of the U-shaped Energy Curve and highly productive.

This fascinating insight lends weight to stress management through self-coaching and also re-perceiving stress as a key to overall energy and vitality management. Stress will excite the orexin system at times that it should not be functioning, specifically bedtime.

Self-coaching is an excellent way to relieve stress and, if done before bed, can actually reduce the activity of the wakefulness neurotransmitter orexin, which can interrupt the sleep that's so vital to our energy. Unlike downing a glass of wine or binging on chocolate, both unhealthy ways to deal with stress, self-coaching goes straight to the source of the problem.

Talking through our problems can reduce our stress hormones, even if that means talking to ourselves. Self-coaching adds some structure to the self-talk, which otherwise can often make things worse as our thoughts wander into predictions and worst-case scenarios. For many people, without some structure or someone else to keep our thinking rational, a disagreement at the office in the morning can become a full-on career crisis by bedtime, in the overactive simulator that is the human mind. Self-coaching will help you to put your thoughts into perspective, thereby reducing your stress-inducing neurotransmitters and paving the way for a sound night's sleep.

So, alas, at this moment there are no orexin hacks for *increasing* wakefulness, but self-coaching offers a great hack for managing orexin and staying within the golden zone of the U-shaped curve. So how to self-coach?

Sometimes we get sucked into the drama of situations that happen in our lives and this is natural, but actually not very useful. If you're unfortunately enough to be lost in the middle of a maze, it would be impossible to see the way out. If, on the other hand, you had the benefit of an aerial view of the maze, and your position in it, it would be much easier for you to find the exit. You can image how stressed you could become stuck in the maze, and how in control you'd feel with benefit of the aerial view. This in essence is the purpose of coaching and why it's an essential skill to keep you in the middle of the Energy Curve, and to reign in any overactive stress hormones and neurotransmitters.

Before we share the 2 golden rules for coaching and the 4 steps involved, we should mention to you that self-coaching is not the same as sports coaching. We often associate coaching with expert advice and "pep-talks," but professional coaching is certainly not that. Self-Coaching and professional coaching are all about observing and acknowledging what's actually happening, and asking the right questions, sometimes the hard questions, to arrive at a solution by yourself. A professional life-coach or executive coach will very rarely give direct advice unless asked to do so or when appropriate, usually towards the end of a session. The best coaches teach people to catch fish by themselves, and we'll teach you how they do it in this section.

The Game with coaching is to think rationally about situations, without emotion and from multiple perspectives, with the goal of reaching the right solution by yourself. The outcome is a feeling of being in-control, motivated and feeling more calm in the process.

The are 2 golden rules with coaching and you can apply them in any life situation too:

Rule #1. Don't get emotionally sucked into the drama of the situation: Observe the situation and your emotions towards it, and then reflect dispassionately, calmly and consider it rationally. You achieve this by taking a satellite level view, not the ground level view.

Rule #2. The second rule is to follow the GROW sequence you will master shortly. GROW stands for Goal, Option, Reality and Will.

Like any game, there are players. The star player who will score the goals and win this game is the pre-frontal cortex (PFC). Remember that this player is so good, it can keep the opposing player, the emotional limbic system, in check, reducing the wakeful activity of orexin that can impact your sleep.

Any great player needs to play in a winning formation and with winning tactics. The sequence we use for self-coaching is the GROW Model of coaching: Goal, Reality, Options, Will. These are the tactics you will use to control the game.

The arena for self-coaching is a quiet space at home where you will not be disturbed for around 20-30 minutes.

GROW Coaching

Once you are sitting quietly and comfortably, you can take a piece of A4 paper and create four sections with space to write your thoughts. The sections are Goal, Reality, Options and Will. The Goal and Will sections can be a little smaller than the Reality and Options sections where you'll do most of the work.

We have created a printable A4 GROW coaching sheet, complete with all of the questions to ask yourself, which you can download at https://motivo-academy/grow-coaching-sheet.

Goal

G is for goal. Without a clear goal, coaching can often go around in circles, a never ending spiral of rumination that will lead to nowhere. So the 1st question you need to ask yourself is, "What is my goal?"

As our objective with self-coaching is to calm our limbic system, a useful approach is to start with the question, "What's happening in my life and how am I doing at the moment? "

Take a few seconds to ponder this question and then focus on a goal. The goal could be, "I would like to feel more in control of this situation," or "I would like to feel more calm right now," or "I would like to make a clear plan to resolve this situation."

Once you have your goal, write it down on the paper in the Goal section.

Reality

R is for Reality. This is the section where you will begin to reflect dispassionately about the situation in question. Before you do this, it's useful to imagine yourself as a satellite looking down at the situation. Remember not to get sucked into the drama of the situation, the limbic system will win that game every time. Your star player, the pre frontal cortex (PFC) works at a satellite level. You're trying to see where you are in the maze and you cannot do that from a ground level perspective. So, from satellite level perspective, explore the "reality" of the situation by asking questions:

- "Tell me more about the situation." Asking yourself this question will start the process of exploring the situation.

- "What's the reason...?" This is your go-to question that you can ask yourself many times to explore the situation in more detail.

- "What emotion do I feel about this situation?" This starts the process of acknowledging your emotions about the situation before calming them. Remember to stay in an observational, satellite level mode and not to get sucked into the drama emotionally. Simply observe your emotions and without feeling them.

- "What's the reason I feel this emotion?" This question helps you to process the emotions you are feeling about the situation so that they can be resolved.

Quick tip: As you answer these questions you will have great insights, write them down. Some may even be options that can go in the Options section.

In our experience as coaches, it can be valuable to put a time limit of 5-10 minutes on exploring the Reality phase. The reason relates to our tendency to ruminate on problems for extended periods of time given the chance. GROW model is effective because it adds a structure to the dialogue and pushes it to a resolution.

After 5-10 minutes, you should feel that you have a much better perspective of the situation. Once you're finished, you can move briskly on to the Options and Obstacles section of the GROW sequence.

Options and Obstacles

As you go through the questions in the Reality section, you'll undoubtedly come across a few good options that will help you to achieve your goal. Options are solutions to your problem and as you think of options, you can write them down on the coaching sheet.

Simply ask yourself the question, "What are my options?"

You want as many options as possible, it's more of a brainstorm than a surgical process. If, "Finding more information on the situation," is an option for your challenge, for example, write that down and move on to other options that may work for you.

Set a time limit of 5-minutes, to write down your options. Coaching should move you briskly towards a logical resolution to the challenge and time constraints will force the best options to surface quickly.

Obstacles are also important to explore in the coaching process. The reason is that many of us already know what we need to do, but our beliefs around the obstacles can hold us back and create mental barriers to resolving our challenges. Simple take 5-minutes to write down the obstacles that are holding you back from achieving your goals and then what you can realistically do to overcome the obstacles. If, "Time," is an obstacle, for example, write it down and what you can do to overcome this obstacle. Maybe you can find one hour late in the afternoon dedicated to achieving your goal.

After 5-10 minutes in the Options and Obstacles section you should feel more in control of your situation, and also have a great list of actions to resolve the challenges. You can now move on to the final section, Will.

Will

Naturally some options will be more effective than others. The final question to ask yourself is, "Of the options I have right now, what will I commit to?" This is the final question to resolve in the GROW model of coaching.

A powerful question that can help in this section, is the, "Gun to the head question." Simply ask yourself, "Gun to the head, what will work?" This is a powerful question that will help you to zone in on exactly what needs to be done, giving your brain the resolution that it needs. Sometimes the option we need to take is the one that we are avoiding, this question will force the best option to the surface.

Once you have chosen the best options that you will commit to, it can be useful to build in a little accountability too. Think about how you will hold yourself accountable to fulfilling the options that you have chosen. How will you reward yourself for achieving it?

Once you've completed the Will section of the GROW sequence, you should now have calmed your emotional limbic system. You star player, the pre frontal cortex (PFC), through it's ability to override the emotional limbic system, should have won the game for you. Emotionally you should be feeling in control of your situation and far less worried.

The tie of day for your self-coaching can be very personal. Although we say to do coaching before bedtime, we don't necessarily recommend it as the last thing you do before sleeping. It can on occasion be more effective earlier in the day. The reason for this is that some people may feel highly energized and excited by the process which can result in a release of dopamine and adrenaline and you may well feel quite "pumped!" If this is the case for you, we encourage you to do your coaching earlier in the day, possibly in the morning before you start work. Once a week if often enough. Its more important that you feel in control of your life and situations and this will have a huge effect on calming your brain and the activity of neurotransmitters such as orexin, which will disrupt your sleep and leave you feeling exhausted and fatigued.

Take the time now to practice self-coaching using the GROW formula. At the end of the exercise, think about what worked and what you can improve next time. Like playing an instrument for the first time, it can take practice you can make it sound great. By taking notes on what you can do to improve your self-coaching technique, you will accelerate your progress dramatically. Apply the improvements in your next session and repeat the process until you become a master coach. This is truly one of the most powerful life changing skills that you can master.

Serotonin

Serotonin is the "happy hormone" which also makes us more awake.[102] Surprisingly, 80% of our serotonin is stored in the gut. It has many functions in the human body, from regulating our bowel movements to helping wounds to heal, and it is crucial to energy and vitality by playing an important role in our mood.

Interestingly, serotonin is behind the butterflies we feel in our stomach. We might get the butterflies waiting to ride a roller coaster, before making a big purchase, while making an important decision, or on a first date.

Flutters in your stomach come from anxiety, excitement, and the thrill that arises from doing something new and unexpected. That is why butterflies fade when you become more familiar with a situation.

These "butterflies" sensations, originate in a network of 100 million neurons lining our stomach and gut, known as our second brain. The size of this mass of neurons is the same as the amount of neurons in a hamster. The brain has too many important things to worry about and delegates digestion to this part of the nervous system. This makes the stomach the only organ able to make decisions without needing the brain. As such, these cells do much more than take care of breaking down food, absorbing nutrients, and expelling waste. They have connections with our brain and play a role in determining our mental state.

Emotions in our brain can trigger a primitive response that causes our stomach to contract. Our brain might feel anxious and it messages this to our gut. At the same time, it triggers the fight-or-flight response by releasing adrenaline, causing our heart rate to rise and sending more blood to our muscles. This means the stomach receives less blood. The second brain doesn't like this and protests to the brain by contracting and making us feel flutters. These contractions are commonly called "butterflies" and have the power to influence our decisions.

The most interesting fact about this second brain is that it hosts 95% of the body's serotonin. This makes your gut a big influencer on your emotions. That is why there is such a huge connection between emotional well-being and gastrointestinal health.

When you experience butterflies in your stomach, it is your serotonin levels changing. It is only when these flutters disappear that your serotonin levels return to normal and you feel happier, calmer, more focused, emotionally stable, and less anxious.

Returning to the brain: more serotonin in the brain means a happier mood but, unfortunately, eating more serotonin does not increase the amount of it in our brain. Serotonin cannot cross the BBB but its precursor, L-tryptophan, an amino acid we associate with sleep, can. Interestingly, most dietary-ingested tryptophan, from bananas, turkey, and other sources, doesn't cross the BBB either.

Amino acids need protein transports to take them over the BBB in the same way that a car needs a ferry to take it across a large body of water.[103] Unfortunately, tryptophan is the least abundant of the amino acids in protein-rich foods, so there is simply too much competition to increase serotonin by dietary means alone. It's not to say, though, that diet doesn't have an impact – because it does.

When we eat carbohydrates, insulin is released, which triggers two things. First, it helps blood sugar to enter cells, and secondly, it facilitates the release of L-tryptophan, which enters the brain to be converted to serotonin. A low-carb diet will affect this. Serotonin has another role to play in the brain: it inhibits dopamine, a neurotransmitter that increases our hunger. Serotonin is also the precursor to melatonin, which helps us to fall asleep each evening.

Serotonin deficiency has also been highly linked to depression.[104] This, too, is very significant. If we remove clinical depression, the clinically significant state of despair and deep sadness, we have other, more subtle and milder types of depression too, such as mild depression and dysthymia. These are more prevalent in women than men. Many can go a lifetime and not know that they have mild depression.

A study of nearly 5000 people in the U.S. concluded that over 20% of those surveyed displayed depressive symptoms, mainly mildly depressive. Even amongst the ones who exhibited severe symptoms, only 38% of those sufferers were getting help.[105]

Without getting into the reasons for depression, which would be a book all of its own, the fact remains that depressed people often lack serotonin in the brain, especially in the amygdala. The usual treatment for depression involves medication called selective serotonin reuptake inhibitors (SSRIs) which inhibit serotonin from being reabsorbed by neurons.[106]

We are certainly not suggesting that SSRIs are a hack for more energy, merely that low serotonin and a "feeling low" mood go hand-in-hand; so maintaining a healthy amount of brain serotonin is a hack for higher vitality. Nonetheless, there are ways to boost serotonin that are safe, natural, and actually work.

Serotonin Hack | Sunlight and Pleasant Memories

Two of the best ways to boost levels of serotonin, in addition to ingesting more L-tryptophan, are exercise and sunlight exposure. In the absence of sun, our body produces extra melatonin. Melatonin regulates the natural sleep cycle. The more melatonin, the sleepier we get. On the other hand, the absence of sun also causes a decrease in the production of serotonin.[107] Sunshine affects the production of serotinin, where the presence of sunlight produces serotonin, and the absence of sunlight not only decreases the production of serotonin, but it increases the production of melatonin. This literally means that on a gray day, we are more susceptible to being sleepy, less happy and therefore less energized. Although we have no control over the weather, it has an effect on us at a chemical level.

If taking a 10-minute walk in the sun is not an option, a sun lamp can be most useful. Being exposed to a 10,000 lux bulb for about 30-minutes per day is enough to improve your mood within two to four days. Light therapy via sun lamps is most effective in the mornings. Having an alarm clock that mimicks the sunrise is also a good way of getting light expsoure even before you wake up. Sometimes called wake up alarm clocks or sunrise alarms, these alarm clocks feature a light that gets gradually brighter after the alarm goes off.

Another way to do increase serotonin is by recalling a pleasant memory. Remembering happy memories can bring back the pleasant feelings tied to the original experience. This has shown to have intrinsic value. During positive reminiscence, there is an engagement of reward-processing and emotion regulation centers and an increase in the release of serotonin. When we recall a memory, we reinforce it in our brain. The more we recall something, the easier it is to recall it in the future. You can think of memories as files in our brain. The more you pull up a file, the easier it is to find it in the future. Like a book that has been read many times, it is easily distinguished from untouched memories. When you remember pleasant memories, you prime your brain to recalling these events. In our daily lives, we encounter many different stimuli. These stimuli activate different memories in our mind. By recalling pleasant memories, we associate elements of our memories to elements that might be found on our daily life. Memories of happy experiences benefit our serotonin production by priming what memories are more susceptible to be recalled by daily triggers. Recalling positive memories, elements that we encounter in our routines will also be charged with a positive halo. This way, our black non-stick frying pan will most likely make us think about a happy morning making pancakes rather than that one time it burnt us. In addition, taking time each day to think about the things in life for which one is grateful can improve serotonin production, and with this happiness and vitality.

These are all excellent ways to stay in the middle of the U-shaped energy curve, as serotonin can be a great mood booster as well as having a calming effect. Beyond how an external factor can affect us biologically, there is a mental and psychological level that we can control. If we are willing to smile, and proactively seek ways to compensate for this external factor, this will affect how we live that day and the amount of vitality we might have. It's how we re-frame our experience that is the key to happiness and vitality.

Dopamine

For the U.S. military, the go-to wakefulness medications for long missions have been amphetamines and a medication called modafinil. Although this is no longer the case, both induce more dopamine in the brain. Dopamine makes you more awake and alert.[108]

Dopamine is an essential neurotransmitter for motivation and reward, especially related to physical activity. In fact, dopamine has an important role in our body movement generally. Parkinson's disease, whose sufferers endure tremors and shaking, have a dysfunctional dopamine system. ADHD is associated with hyperexcitability as well. Studies have shown that medications that help to regulate the dopamine system help to alleviate its symptoms too.[109]

Dopamine makes us feel more alert and awake and benefits working memory too. This is due to the large number of dopamine receptors in the prefrontal cortex (PFC). The frontal cortex hosts the reward system pathway, which is the corner stone of motivation. This system runs on dopamine. The prefrontal cortex is also very involved in selecting which stimuli from the world we process consciously. Although our brain processes incredible amounts of information, only a very small percentage of it is available to us on a conscious level. Because the frontal lobe of the cerebral cortex is largely in charge of motivation, it relies on our goals to select which stimuli are worth processing with more detail. Having healthy levels of dopamine assures you take in all the information you need to purposefully meet your goals."

Interestingly, a study has confirmed that a particular type of meditation called Yoga Nidra, which is associated with a reduced readiness for action, resulted in a 62% increase in dopamine release.[110]

The goal with dopamine is to keep it in the middle of the energy curve, not too much and not too little. Too much dopamine can make us feel over stimulated and once its depleted can induce anxiety. Too little dopamine can make us feel fatigued and listless but we need to boost it in healthy and productive ways. One of the best ways is to learn to master the art of goal setting once and for all.

Dopamine Hack | Mastering the Short-Term Goal/Reward Cycle

Humans have many ways to motivate behavior. One of the most effective is by triggering the reward system. Setting short-term goals and achieving them is rewarding in itself. This is because it activates the dopamine system. This system is regulated by the amygdala, dopamine system, and the striatal system. The brain spots an opportunity and accesses the memory to determine if it's a threat or potentially rewarding. If it's potentially rewarding, the brain releases dopamine, which energizes us to take positive action. If the opportunity is associated with disappointment, dopamine is not released and we are not energized to take action. The genius of the system is that once we take action, the brain determines if it was worth the energy, in what psychologists call the "reward prediction error." If the brain thinks it was worth the energy, there is another activation of the dopamine system, which in turn informs the striatal system. The function of the striatal system is to update your memory so that you know for future reference what gives reward and what doesn't, i.e., where we should expend our energy and where we shouldn't.

Choose goals that are in line with your values, a long-term vision that inspires you, and the things that you love doing. Take a piece of paper and a pen and write a list of five goals that you could achieve (with some effort required) within the next two weeks. Make them goals that you know you will find rewarding. Then choose one, the one that will give you the greatest satisfaction, maybe the most challenging one or the one that will give you the biggest result. According to its level of difficulty, think about an appropriate reward: an ice cream, something that you want, maybe a movie at the cinema, etc.

Next, make a plan to achieve the goal and focus all of your energy on achieving it. Do not allow yourself to be distracted. When you have achieved your goal, celebrate and reward yourself. Importantly, enjoy that feeling of achievement for at least 24 hours. Both adrenaline and dopamine will give you an energizing boost and they will reinforce the habit of winning. The key is the period of celebrating, called the "consumption period." This period of allowing yourself to enjoy your victory and reward is vital, neurologically, for habit forming.

Finally, update your list of goals and set another one. Repeat the process. Repeating the process will hack the dopamine system once again and give you the energizing boost and motivated feeling that you're looking for.

Adrenaline and Noradrenaline

Adrenaline sports conjure up images of skydiving and bungee jumping. Adrenaline (sometimes called epinephrine) is secreted by the adrenal glands and cannot pass the blood brain barrier (BBB), while noradrenaline (also called norepinephrine) is synthesized and stored in the brain, where it is used as a neurotransmitter. Both have an important role to play in our survival. They form a part of the famed "fight, flight or freeze" response. At times of perceived danger, neurons begin to release noradrenaline.

The adrenal glands start releasing their own epinephrine and pumping it into the bloodstream, which causes a response fit for an altercation with a tiger or a public speaking engagement. Our blood vessels tighten and our airways relax and dilate considerably, helping us to take on more oxygen. Meanwhile, the liver begins to pump glucose into the bloodstream and converts glycogen, stored glucose, back into glucose. This prepares us for any reaction we might take.

So why is adrenaline important for energy?

Adrenaline will certainly give you a hit of energy, of that there is no question. More oxygen is inhaled and glucose released, but it's not much use for anything other than exercise and running away from tigers and hostile audiences. The problem is that adrenaline is vasoconstrictive, meaning that it tightens blood vessels. Also, brain functions of the prefrontal cortex (PFC), the thinking part of the brain, are limited in their action when noradrenaline is too high.[111] Just a little is helpful to the PFC, which has a very large number of connections with adrenaline-releasing neurons, but too much is not helpful.[112]

So adrenaline will boost your energy and move you to the right hand side of the U-shaped Energy Curve we looked at earlier. If you are at the low end of the Energy Curve, adrenaline will move you towards the productive middle zone. Too much time at the stressed end of the Energy Curve, however, is damaging to our health as prolonged exposure to adrenaline can be detrimental. According to the American Psychological Association, stress can lead to Type 2 diabetes, infertility in both men and women, increased cholesterol, high blood pressure, heart attack, and stroke.

Now, there is something essential we should know. The way we think about stress has an effect on how stress itself affects us. A very interesting study had participants watch one of either two videos. One video talked about stress as a performance enhancer and the other one talked about stress as hurtful to performance. It was interesting to find that the participants who saw stress as beneficial did much better at a mock interview given after watching the video. What was really interesting was that saliva samples were taken from participants. Those who watched the video which showed stress as a performance enhancer released neurosteroids, which counter the effects of cortisol, another hormone involved in our stress response. By adjusting our mindset and seeing stress as an enhancing mechanism, we can gain an advantage out of it.[113] This leads us to our first hack for adrenaline.

Adrenaline Hack (Decrease) | Re-perceive Stress as a Friend

Changing how you think about stress can actually make you healthier by changing your bodily response to stress. For example, when we believe stress signs like: pounding heart and faster breathing, are physical changes that prepare us to perform better at a task by supplying more blood to our brain and delivering more oxygen, the way our blood vessels react shifts. When we see stress as a positive bodily function, our blood vessels don't contract and, on the contrary, stay relaxed, even though our heart keeps beating fast. This looks a lot like what happens when we experience joy and happiness. The reason why chronic stress is associated with heart problems is because of this blood vessel contraction. It is not healthy to have your blood vessels tight and small. But, on the other hand, having a fast heart beat with relaxed veins correlates with healthy aging.[114] This is the very essence of what it is to feel vitalized, stimulated and energized. To experience the high energy and focus without anxiety or fear.

The idea is not to get rid of stress, but to make sure we use it to our advantage. Stress is a way your body helps you rise to a challenge. A very interesting study followed 30,000 adults for 8 years. They asked them how much stress they had experienced in the past year and they also asked how harmful they thought stress was. People who experience a lot of stress had a 43% higher risk of dying in the next year, but this was only true for those who believed stress was bad for them. The people who experienced a lot of stress but did not consider stress harmful had the lowest "death expectancy" rate out of all the groups, even compared to those who experienced little to no stress.[115]

Adrenaline is also important for memories, especially fear-related ones, which trigger its response.[116] A feature of the adrenaline response is the release of glucose, which increases brain functions related to memory storage.[117]

Norepinephrine, which is primarily used in the brain, is essential for working memory and attention processes. In fact, norepinephrine and dopamine work together for optimal functioning. Nonetheless, excessive amounts of either of them are counterproductive.[118] Too much dopamine, epinephrine, and norepinephrine would hinder productivity and place you on the far right side of the U-shaped Energy Curve.

The energy hack with adrenaline is daily practice at re-perceiving stress as performance enhancing and energy boosting. A good approach here is to spend 5-minutes answering the self-reflective questions:

"Where is the stress in my life right now, how can I use it, what skill do I need to learn in order to adapt and overcome the challenge, this stress is pushing me to a better place, where might that be?"

Start now by taking 5 minutes to answer those questions now.

Adrenaline Hack (Increase) | Put Yourself in Stretch

So, noradrenaline is important for cognitive performance, but it's also responsible for feeling fear. Noradrenaline and dopamine go hand in hand; in fact, *both* are needed for effective working memory and cognitive functions – in moderation. Psychologists have known something for a very long time: humans are intrinsically motivated towards learning and progress. Learning, along with the accompanying sense of progression, is considered to be essential for the happiness of both children and adults. Learning, perhaps unsurprisingly, also prevents dementia.

Progression entails leaving your comfort zone, which by definition means experiencing and facing our fears. Too much fear results in panic, too little fear results in stagnation.

Nature has hardwired us to enjoy the vitality, the subjective energy, of feeling truly alive through the dopamine-norepinephrine partnership in the PFC. Think how great you feel when you do something that initially scares you, like riding a rollercoaster or nailing an important presentation.

The hack is to keep your dopamine and norepinephrine levels in the middle of the Energy Curve by consistently being in stretch and challenging yourself to do new and exciting things, to face your fears, to go to new places, to learn and then practice new skills, and most of all, to have fun doing so. This is not only borne out in the science, it's one of the most frequently observed traits in successful people with high vitality.

Good examples include visiting somewhere new and exciting, even just trying a new cuisine you've never eaten before. It could go as far as climbing a mountain, trying scuba or surfing for the first time, going for a personal best, applying for a more senior job, getting critical feedback or public speaking to a slightly bigger audience. Whatever it is for you, make it a daily practice to spend time in stretch, outside of your comfort zone. The word "stretch" is important, it means to not too comfortable, but also not to reach to far into a "panic" zone.

Remember to always re-perceive any stress or anxiety you feel in the stretch zone as health motivational stress that's energizing and pushing you to a better place in your life.

Take a few minutes now, to write down a list of challenges that would take you out of your comfort zone. Once you have your list, choose one or two to commit to and then make plan and set a deadline to achieve them. Happy stretching!

Brain-Derived Neurotrophic Factor

A growing body of evidence is highlighting the importance of the brain-derived neurotrophic factor (BDNF) as one of the key factors to understanding energy and neuroplasticity, the brain's ability to change and grow. BDNF is a crucial neurotransmitter/protein in the brain which regulates glucose and energy metabolism.

Researchers from the University of California, Los Angeles (UCLA) showed that BDNF prevents the decay of neurons and that BDNF can be significantly controlled by exercise.[119] That means that exercise has a large positive impact on BDNF levels in the brain.[120][121]

More BDNF equals more energy. Indeed, the research suggests not only that BDNF levels can be increased with exercise, but for individuals who have a previous history of high-level athletic exercise, a much less frequent amount of exercise is required to elicit the same amount of BDNF secretion.

One of the most interesting discoveries is from brain scans using fMRI scans and EEG. They were used to determine the strength of electrical signals in specific areas of the brain for test subjects based on their levels of exercise. Researchers made a startling discovery: not only did exercise increase energy levels, but specific types of exercise were associated with higher energy levels in specific regions of the brain. In particular, exercise which incorporated complex movements, such as martial arts, increased electrical signal strength in the PFC, the area of the brain responsible for goals, planning, working memory, retrieval and which can also regulate the amygdala.[122]

Why is this important? The amygdala, as we know, governs the "fight, flight, or freeze" response and is often inaccurate in judging threats and rewards from a distance. Its proximity to the hippocampus, which stores long-term memories (especially emotional ones), is no accident. The amygdala determines threats and potential issues and orders the release of adrenaline if needed. The amygdala errs on the side of caution to keep you alive; threats encountered in the wild are often from predators, and our natural predators are often very quick. If the human brain had to deliberate every life-saving reaction, our species would have died off long ago. Dangerous predators fortunately no longer surround most of us, but unfortunately, our amygdala hasn't evolved to that reality and is still highly reactive for many people. This causes anxiety and stress, propelling us to the wrong end of the U-shaped Energy Curve.

The PFC is our savior here. The wise and thoughtful PFC can actually regulate the sensitive amygdala. This is the neuropsychological basis for any type of therapy, especially cognitive behavioral therapy (CBT). The PFC thinks while the amygdala just reacts, and higher levels of energy in the PFC can only be a good thing. Complex movement cardio can increase BDNF in the PFC, which in turn could help to keep your cognition sharp yet less reactive.

So complex movement cardio such as martial arts or boxing is a BDNF hack for greater energy and energy regulation. A true fatigue fighter which we strongly recommend.

A quick reminder: trans fats negatively affect the amount of BDNF in the brain, which then relates to less energy. Avoid trans fats at all costs to keep your energy in the golden zone of the U-shaped Energy Curve.

BDNF Hack | Complex Movement Cardio

Grizzly autopsy images placed on cigarette packages are evidence that people really have a short-term motivation, as in most countries the tactic has been ineffective at getting smokers to quit. The packages serve merely to scare your kids when they go to the store and do little to motivate smokers to kick the habit.[123] Human nature, it would seem, motivates us to act on the short term and not the longer term.

We feel that by marketing the long-term benefits of cardio exercise, public health marketers and other proponents of this type of exercise are missing one of its greatest benefits: higher energy and vitality, whose effects on the body are almost immediate. Whatever happened to exercising just to feel great?

Few of us work in a physically demanding environment, yet our mental energy is heavily influenced not only by our diets but also our exercise habits. Exercise actually increases BDNF, which regulates energy metabolism in the brain, and boosts ghrelin as well as AMPK, which as you learned earlier helps you to learn and is important for mitochondrial biogenesis. Mitochondrial biogenesis is the process of adding more of the energy producing mitochondria in your body which happens during exercise and in cold temperatures.

Cardio increases your brain energy. A report by researchers Fernando Gomez-Pinilla and Chris Hillman at UCLA indicated the astounding benefits of cardio exercise on brain energy, especially in the area of the brain associated with decisions and goals, the mighty pre frontal cortex (PFC). Using an EEG, they measured what's known as P3 latency to track the time between a stimulus and the time it takes to register in a specific brain region representing your conscious mind. They also measured the strength of the wave. A low latency is a sign of good brain health and quick reaction times. The researchers found that the P3 waves from EEG tests were much stronger and had lower latency in those who exercised regularly than those who didn't. That means that the brain responded to a stimulus quicker and with more power, requiring less processing time.[124] This is an incredible finding which shows that cardiovascular exercise truly enhances your cognition.

Exercise actually up-regulates the amount of energy in the brain, and not the other way round. Gomez and Pinilla said in their report that: "It is significant that exercise regulates elements by which the body signals the brain about aspects of energy homeostasis (the body's ability to maintain a constant supply of energy) that are crucial for regulation of cognitive function... especially learning."

Incredibly, further studies have revealed that different types of exercise can increase BDNF in specific regions of the brain. For example, complex movement exercise increases the amount of BDNF and therefore energy in the PFC. Rhythmic exercise associated with meditative body scanning, such as running, increases BDNF in the amygdala and hippocampus. But in a study between taekwondo, running, boxing, taekwondo came out on top for increasing BDNF.[125] Other studies comparing running to martial arts have shown that it was the latter that improved functioning in the PFC, although all exercise can increase information-processing speed.[126]

The benefits of exercise for mental energy can be enjoyed in just a few weeks. In fact, for those who previously had a habit of exercise, it requires less exercise to elicit the same response. Unfortunately for those just starting to hit the gym for the first time, it may require a little more effort. Nonetheless the results are real and will happen quickly. You *will* feel great.

The added benefit of cardio is that it helps your body to use glucose without the use of insulin, and this unique effect happens for around two hours after exercise. For those looking to lose weight, the optimal time to eat carbohydrates, therefore, is just after exercise. The positive effects on insulin sensitivity last for around 16 hours. Although insulin is also essential for the brain, as we saw with the diet hacks, increasing both cognitive performance and also memory function, we need to be sparing with it in order to maintain insulin sensitivity and avoid insulin resistance. Insulin resistance is most definitely associated with fatigue, low energy and low vitality.[127]

Exercise also increases dopamine, which plays a key role in reward/motivation, learning, and the feeling of energy, vitality, and motivation. Higher amounts of dopamine and BDNF will mean better physical and mental well-being as well as effective learning.

In our corporate training work, we start training sessions with a 1-minute shadow boxing workout followed by a breathing routine. The aim is to activate noradrenaline, dopamine, BDNF, and AMPK and to bring the trainees into the middle of the Energy Curve for optimal performance. The increase in cerebral blood flow is the boost that many participants need to wake up and get engaged. Our experience is that learning increases and participants have more energy during training sessions when these types of exercises precede training.

Although most leaders would be considered oddball for requiring their staff to do a minute of shadow boxing before work, many businesses do offer subsidized gym memberships as a benefit – although the trend has dwindled in recent years. The main reason for companies to offer gym memberships is often simply the wellness and long-term health of their employees. Companies should also consider that gym memberships can offer a performance advantage too, by increasing cerebral blood flow and the activity of the performance boosting neurotransmitters and proteins in their employees.

One of our favorite hacks for an immediate energy boost at any time of day is a 1-minute shadow boxing or jogging on the spot routine. An interesting study conducted on sleep-deprived women showed that stair walking was more energizing than a small dose of caffeine.[128] Again, a very simple hack that can be part of everyone's daily routine: simply take the stairs and not the elevator (unless you work on the 50th floor of course).

Ghrelin

We could not write a book about human energy without writing about ghrelin which, surprisingly, was only identified in 1999. Ghrelin is a hormone that is mostly released from the stomach and it's critically important for managing energy homeostasis, i.e., making sure you have enough energy.[129]

Ghrelin motivates you to eat (it's the "hungry hormone"), and its cousin, leptin, is the "I'm full hormone." When ghrelin is released into the bloodstream, it signals to the brain to look for food. It works closely with the dopamine system and even has receptors in the ventral tegmental area of the brain, which is your dopamine center. Remember, the dopamine system is the one that increases our appetite in the presence of food and is responsible for reward.[130]

In fact, the system has evolved so that we are motivated to find food especially when it is scarce, but also when it is not scarce; this causes us to put on weight, just in case of a future famine. We do, however, live in an age when we are just a click away from food. Ghrelin and the behaviors that it motivates may explain our tendency to yo-yo between under-eating and overeating when we are on diets. Your body simply doesn't want or need a six-pack, no matter how much your conscious mind desires one.

Ghrelin is released into the system at numerous times of day and in a variety of ways: when blood glucose is low, when norepinephrine is higher and also when the brain anticipates food. Incredibly, when our stomach stretches, ghrelin stops being released and leptin is released instead.[131]

Crucially for vitality, ghrelin influences orexin, the "wakeful hormone:" more ghrelin means more orexin. The effect that the release of ghrelin has on the body is profound and, according to researchers at Munich University, includes "the stimulation of appetite, lipid accumulation, the modulation of immunity and inflammation, the stimulation of gastric motility, the improvement of cardiac performance, the modulation of stress, anxiety, taste sensation and reward-seeking behavior, as well as the regulation of glucose metabolism and thermogenesis."[132] That's quite a list!

Why do we eat more at times of stress? Researchers from MIT may have the answer. The researchers were interested in why sufferers of PTSD didn't always show biomarkers from the hypothalamus-pituitary-adrenal axis (HPA), the parts of the brain responsible for the fight-flight-freeze response. The research implicated increases in ghrelin and its derivative growth hormone (GH) acting on the amygdala to facilitate the learned fear we associate with PTSD.

It seems that stress eating could be a protective behavior to prevent long-term psychological damage (by lowering ghrelin). The increase in ghrelin activity in the amygdala could, as a side effect, modify our feeding and eating behavior whilst the learning and encoding is happening. This could be used as a warning sign that we are, at that moment, affecting our long-term mental health.[133]

Our hack for gherlin is not to increase it, you don't need to generate the feeling of extra hunger, but to be attuned to it. When you are feeling hungry, drink water and then make sure you are ingetsing all the nutrients your body needs. Maybe a large meal is not always necessary and a small nutritious snack will be enough. Eat accordingly. Your body has evolved to tell you when it needs nutrients, making you more alert. This lends weight to ghrelin having an important role in our feelings of alertness.[134] Nonetheless, when hunger becomes too intense, this alertness will come at the expense of impairing cognition and focus. In other words it will become a distraction and not a valuable friend to your feelings of wellbeing and vitality.

Neuro Hack 5 | Stimulants

Caffeine

Humanity has embraced the caffeinated drink as its stimulant of choice. Coffee is an energizer, no doubt about it. Nonetheless, too much coffee can overstimulate, leaving a slightly anxious, "bouncing-off-the-walls" kind of energy which leads to a significant dip afterwards. Let's take a closer look at the world's most popular stimulant and decide if, and how much to take.

Coffee is a worldwide favorite. It is one of the top five most consumed drinks across the globe due to its delicious and bitter yet smooth aroma. We love the texture and the little perk it gives us in the morning. Make no mistake, caffeine works for us. Coffee is already probably the most common energy hack in your toolkit – but there are some cons to weigh against the pros. It's wise to read on to make a balanced decision about how much you should lean on coffee versus some of the alternatives.

Yes, coffee works for us, yet we find that sustaining our energy levels purely on caffeine is somewhat counterproductive. After three or four cups of the stuff, many of us get pretty cranky, start multiple different tasks, and fail to complete any of them. We're working harder all right, but not much work is actually getting done. Also, we find that after 4 p.m., when we know we shouldn't drink coffee, we have very little to keep us going at a time of day when we need a steady, consistent, calm release of powerful energy in order to get to the finish.

There are times when we feel like we need to be an industrial robot with the speed of a jet and the agility of a fly while staying calm and Zen-like. Although we may get the first part of that equation, the calm and Zen-like component is often lacking after drinking coffee, and in truth we can often end up feeling slightly anxious. So what's the science behind this?

Adenosine, as we have seen, is a neurotransmitter which makes us feel gradually more sleepy throughout the day and it also suppresses the central nervous system (CNS). Caffeine is cunning, it prevents adenosine from doing its job because it sits on the adenosine receptor of the cell. Imagine a helicopter with nowhere to land because there's a bus parked on the helipad.

Without the suppressant effect of adenosine to hold back the activity of neurons, the neuron continues to become more excited, a bit like a nuclear reactor with the control rods drawn up.

Adenosine also has a key role in vasodilation (healthy widening of the arteries), which, amongst other functions, helps the body to clear toxins from the brain as we sleep. In addition, if we have not slept well, and our brains are still chock-full of neurotoxins, our choice of caffeine the next day could be the worst possible choice for brain health. As we have seen, neurotoxins are cleared from the brain through convection processes aided by vasodilation. The evidence does not yet exist to suggest that neurotoxins are cleared while we are awake. Adenosine is our ally in this process: once adenosine receptors have been occupied by the caffeine molecules and the cell becomes more excited, the pituitary gland begins to instruct the adrenal glands to release adrenaline, which, as we have seen, isn't necessarily the hormone we want for mental focus on complex tasks, although in small doses it is useful.

Again, for energy, we are really looking for something a little more smooth, purposeful, powerful, and calm, and a little less haphazard and "Geronimo." Without question, if you have not slept the night before, coffee if going to make you feel more awake; but too much of it could be hurting your brain at this sensitive time.

There's plenty of evidence to suggest some improvements in reaction times and cognitive performance, but one study stands out for its counterargument: that, although there are some cognitive enhancements, they aren't always beneficial. This finding perfectly captures our view on caffeine.

An intriguing study from the University of Vienna found evidence that caffeine hinders certain activities requiring high functioning cognition, such as chess.[135]

The researchers put together a trial in which they pitted tournament chess players versus computers, with each human player doped with caffeine, modafinil, methylphenidate, or a placebo. The results were surprising. The scores of the doped players were actually worse than the one who took the placebo. Why was this? The researchers noted that the doped players took much longer over their moves and were being penalized for missing the time limits the game imposes for each move. Their depth of processing may have improved but they may also have been distracted. Their their lack of self-control in sticking to the all-important time limits meant that they would have been better off without the stimulants.

The International Chess Federation, which believe it or not has a list of banned substances (which includes modafinil and methylphenidate), had excluded caffeine from their list, so the effects are not considered a major benefit on the cognitive front.

Caffeine works by restricting adenosine activity, which in turn creates an excitatory response. Those receptors are mainly found in the high-functioning "thinking" part of the brain, our friend the pre frontal cortex (PFC), which is why we get a slight boost in cognition. However, caffeine's excitatory effects simply stimulate *everything* in the PFC.[136] Caffeine is more of an energy grenade than a precision instrument.

Research also suggests tea as a great energy source. Tea has a soothing component called L-theanine. L-theanine is often used for anxiety as it can induce feelings of calm without drowsiness and it also reduces blood pressure.[137] It is shown that one strong espresso or six cups of black tea (astoundingly, the same amount of caffeine, at 184 mg) *reduced* cerebral blood flow by an astounding 20% and 21% respectively.[138] Another study from Taiwan concluded that black tea increases cerebral blood flow;[139] and yet another study showed that tea in fact reverses the vasoconstrictive (tightening of arteries) effects of coffee, yet also noted that any mood or cognitive performance-enhancing effects were lost.[140]

Caffeine, as we have seen, increases blood pressure and is a vasoconstrictor, which is not generally good for cognitive function as the brain needs a good supply of glucose and oxygen from the bloodstream. One imagines how much more effective caffeine would be if it didn't have that downside characteristic. Tea could be the best answer, as it contains both caffeine and L-theanine to balance the effects.[141]

In addition to being loaded with antioxidants, tea has cognitive enhancing properties. L-theanine increases alpha waves, which are associated with feelings of calm and relaxation. The amounts found in tea enhance brain activity. When caffeine is consumed through coffee, it improves concentration and alertness.[142]

One study confirmed that L-theanine and caffeine, taken together, have clear beneficial effects on sustained attention, memory, and suppression of distraction. Moreover, L-theanine was found to lead to relaxation by reducing "caffeine induced arousal." [143]

So, what's the takeaway here? Caffeine is personal. Your choice of coffee or tea comes down to your own sensitivity and your own personal attitude. Many people grab a coffee out of habit or in desperation to stay focused. Your aim is to consciously stay within the middle of the U-shaped Energy Curve for an enjoyable vitality that's also productive and therefore good for your motivation and self-esteem. If coffee helps with that, then it's the right tool for you right now, but just being aware of the alternatives is an energy hack in itself. Your brain may simply need to focus on something different for fifteen minutes so it's worth trying a break before reaching for the espresso.

Tea has the benefit of helping you to stay calmer and of not being vasoconstrictive, unlike coffee. Caffeine of any description can interrupt your sleep, however; so coffee, which is naturally higher in caffeine, should be limited to the morning time.

For some readers, the ideal solution for you could be to avoid the stimulant altogether. One minute of cardio will increase cerebral blood flow and has the same impact as a cup of coffee without the side effects, so it's an excellent alternative in the late afternoon or early evening. This is one of our favorite hacks prior to writing in the evening.

Modafinil

Modafinil, marketed as Provigil in the U.S., has been prescribed for narcolepsy sufferers for many years. This chemical stimulant was developed by the Defense Advanced Research Projects Agency (DARPA), an agency of the U.S. Department of Defense responsible for the development of emerging technologies for use by the military. This drug is the only approved wakefulness medication used by the U.S. Air Force and has been assessed by many armed forces globally. In the U.S., however, modafinil is a prescription-only medication and has some side effects in around 30% of users.

According to the manufacturer these can include anxiety and headaches. Although the mechanism for its effectiveness was not immediately clear when the drug was introduced, it now seems that the drug acts on the dopamine system as a dopamine reuptake inhibitor, increasing the amount of dopamine in the system in the same way that cocaine, Ritalin, or psychotropic drugs work. For that very reason, it has been added to a list of controlled substances and is not regularly prescribed or recommended for healthy people.

We don't recommend using Modafinil to fight fatigue and to feel more energized, but we felt that some of our readers may be considering it as an option. Medications, are always a very last resort especially considered the huge number of alternatives which require only minor changes to your diet and the exercises and habits you've learned in this chapter. We are very confident that if you can follow the advice in this book, you should never need to medicate to feel more energy and vitality in your life

Summary

The foundation of balancing neurotransmitters is having enough of them to begin with. That means getting a sufficient protein intake that includes many protein sources (including vegetables). The next step is controlling fermented foods and drinks so that you can get enough of the wakefulness neurotransmitter L-histidine.

The golden zone of the U-shaped Energy Curve is your target, and our neuro-hacks can help you get there. You can increase your motivation neurotransmitters dopamine and noradrenaline with L-tyrosine supplementation and setting rewarding "stretch" goals for yourself.

If you have too much energy, the calming effects of serotonin can be hacked with exercise, recall of a pleasant memory, and sunlight, with L-tryptophan supplementation. You can also re-perceive stress as a friend and teacher, which will help you to move back into the productive middle zone.

The wakefulness neurotransmitters ghrelin and orexin can be increased by not eating between meals. Self-coaching before bed will calm levels of orexin, which interrupt sleep.

Balancing your personal Energy Curve is an exercise in continuous awareness of where your energy levels are in that moment, are you too stressed, under-stimulated or just right. Act on that awareness, use the hacks in this section to maintain that middle zone. This will take conscious effort at first but will become a habit in time. Your body naturally wants to be in the middle zone, you can help it and work with your physiology to achieve it.

Once your energy is in the productive middle zone then shoot for the efficiency hacks in this section to help you take full advantage of it.

MOTIVATIONAL ENERGY

So far in this book we have looked at physiological ways to increase vitality from the perspectives of our basic biology and more complex neuroscience. But there is yet another facet of energy that every book on this topic should mention: human motivation. We've all found ourselves doing things we are not fully committed to. Imagine dancing to a song you are just not into, writing a report on a topic you detest, or cooking something quickly because you're hungry. All of these activities in themselves have the potential to trigger a very different motivational response. Now imagine that *your* song comes up at a party, you're writing a report on a topic you are incredibly interested in, or you are taking a cooking class with your favorite chef. Our motivation and will to invest our energy on specific activities has a large and direct impact on our energy levels. Indeed, a loss of motivation has a huge impact on feelings of fatigue and burnout. Conversely, it can be the fastest way to experience higher feelings of energy and vitality.

Two very broad motivators are success and happiness. These motivators are what connects each and every one of us. Remember this the next time you are on a crowded commuter train. Despite the fact that we all share those same two motivators, many of us tend to stick to safety instead. As you compete for every inch of space on the crowded station platform, try to remember that at our core we strive together for the same motivations. Indeed, the Latin origins of the word, "compete," derives from, "To strive and grow together."

We can essentially define motivation as the desire to act and invest our energy towards a specific objective, whether it is going to the fridge to find a snack or running away from a wild bear. We are motivated to achieve a desired state or an unmet need, whether it is safety or satiety, feeling loved or feeling mastery, self-esteem or relaxation.

The motivation side of energy is about the power of the mind. Until now, we have seen what goes on in the brain and what goes on in the body. Now we will focus on our subjective experience of life, our goals, our battles, and our ability to align all of the aspects in our lives to achieve the emotional state we experience as vitality

One example of the effect of a lack of motivation on vitality is burnout. Usually when we burnout we experience a physical and psychological exhaustion and it often involves a sense of reduced accomplishment and loss of personal identity. Burnout can result from various factors, including:

1) Work-life imbalance: If your work takes up so much of your time and effort that you don't have the energy to spend time with family and friends or doing the things that help your to refresh.

2) Extremes of activity: A monotonous or chaotic profession, maybe a job that requires constant energy to remain focused.

3) Lack of control: Feeling the absence of influence on decisions that affect your job — such as your schedule, assignments or workload.

4) Unclear job expectations: If you're unclear about what is expected from you, on workload or authority.

5) Dysfunctional workplace dynamics: Finding yourself in a toxic environment, undermined by colleagues or having a boss that micromanages your work.

6)Lack of social support: Feeling isolated at work and in your personal life.

Although many times burnout can be addressed in the short term by taking some time off, at the end of the day the issue will only be resolved by addressing the core issues and understanding your motivation and deeper purpose in regards to your choice of job.

Motivation has been well studied in psychology for over 100 years. There are many strong theories that have evolved over time, adding to our understanding of what compels us to take action. One of the most famous psychologists to propose a theory of motivation was Abraham Maslow. In 1943 Maslow proposed that motivation was the pursuit of what he called, "unmet needs."

Maslow described several levels of human needs that are common to most people throughout their lives and placed them in a hierarchy visually represented on a pyramid which he called the "Hierarchy of needs." (see illustration page 112). He identified the needs as basic needs, survival needs, social needs, esteem needs, and at the very top of the pyramid, the need for self-actualization. To self-actualize is to realize your true potential. In Maslow's original theory of the hierarchy of needs, the levels were sequential, with one level needing to be completely satisfied for the next to be the motivator: i.e., you can't be immediately motivated to reach your true potential if you don't yet have self-esteem. Maslow's levels are an excellent basic framework to help identify the main motivators in our lives, and where there may be a gap.

Knowing and pursuing the need in your life that serves as your immediate motivation helps your brain to avoid what's known as, cognitive dissonance. Cognitive dissonance is the feeling we get when holding two opposing views, especially when we know that what we are doing could be wrong. We often experience cognitive dissonance as a feeling of guilt. The hierarchy of Needs is valuable because the brain always knows that it has problems to resolve and needs to be met. When we procrastinate from meeting those needs by pursuing lower priority tasks, we feel a sense of unease. Knowing our priority motivator allows us to set goals and take actions that are in alignment that are in line with our immediate needs. We can call this alignment, "Cognitive consonance," which is one of the most valuable energy hacks in this book.

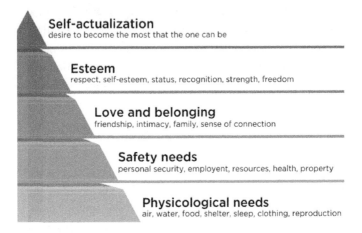

Look at the hierarchy of needs pyramid shown above. Which of your needs have you already satisfied, and which are unmet? Start at the bottom and work your way up until you have identified your unmet need. This need is your priority motivator. With your priority motivator in mind, you can now set a goal and a strategy to address this need.

Your strategy will need to be broken into tasks and added as priorities to your to-do list. If, for example, your needs are satisfied up until the self-actualization level, write down a strategy for how you will express your true potential and self-actualize. The strategy could include making a business plan for a new business or seeking a new job to reach the next level in your career. The associated tasks on your to-do list could include buying a book on writing a business plan or sending your CV to a headhunter. This priority motivator is the place to invest your energy.

The hierarchy is a valuable guide that can help you to define your goals, strategies, plans, and daily actions which we also use in our coaching work in the order he originally prescribed.

When we satisfy and unmet need, we activate the reward system and release dopamine. As we learned in the past section on dopamine, the brain spots a possible opportunity and predicts the chances of an adequate reward for the investment of our precious energy. Once we have achieved the goal, the brain goes into consumption mode and decides if it was worth all the effort. If it was satisfying and worth the effort the dopamine system lights up like a Christmas tree. The striatal neurons get the message to update our learning centers in the prefrontal cortex (PFC), and hippocampus and our behavior are changed accordingly. If we were not satisfied and it wasn't worth the effort, the dopamine system is as quiet as a mouse, and there is no positive reinforcement for future behavior.

As with any substance that induces a dopamine response, by consistently identifying and satisfying your unmet needs, achievement can become addictive and habitual. Focusing on pursuing beneficial unmet needs identified using Maslow's heirarchy is a healthy habit we can all benefit from. The key is to allow yourself the consumption time to savor your victory, using the dopamine system for its naturally intended purpose. Your brain will thank you for it, and your energy levels will thank you too.

Building this practice into your daily or weekly routine will produce the greatest rewards over time.

Motivation Hack 1 | Challenge your Beliefs: Why You Don't Achieve Your Goals

Think about your priority unmet need on the hierarchy of needs. Now answer this question: Why have you not yet satisfied that need?

It's one thing to know your priority need, it's quite another to satisfy it. Although there might be many reasons that come to mind when answering that question, one important factor you might have not considered is your underlying belief system.

Sometimes it's what we believe about the things that we want that can hold us back from achieving them. Some beliefs can give us the confidence to achieve our goals, and other beliefs can hold us back. If you believe that you won't be accepted into a university for example, that belief may dent your commitment to writing a successful application or even put you off from applying at all. These beliefs are called limiting beliefs.

When it comes to motivation, beliefs are analogous to a swimmer holding a huge rock under water. The rock (i.e., a limiting belief) holds the swimmer under the surface. However, if the swimmer can drop the rock, they can float effortlessly to the surface. If you can drop your limiting beliefs about your priority need, you will remove at least some of the mental obstacles that could be holding you back from achieving it.

Many people fail to achieve their next level because of a belief they hold about that level. A common example is the "love and belonging" need. Some people who have this need, yet have failed to satisfy it often hold limiting beliefs such as, "I can't be loved," or, "I loved someone once and it didn't work out." These limiting beliefs can then prevent them from trying to meet new people or taking their chances in a new relationship.

If "esteem" is your priority need, you may hold a limiting belief such as, "I'm just not that good at anything," or, "other people are luckier than I am." These limiting beliefs may prevent you from doing the things that could boost your self esteem such as applying for a promotion or learning and mastering a new skill.

With needs that you struggle to satisfy, there is almost always a limiting belief to go with it. It's certainly not the only factor, there are often very real logistical and practical limitations on what we can achieve, however our blocks are often mental and our limiting beliefs are often unfounded. Nothing saps your energy more than a feeling of resignation, and few things are as tragic as potential that was wasted because of mistaken beliefs.

Understanding our deeply held beliefs about ourselves and the world around is a challenge for most people. With fast paced lives and a natural inclination in all people towards self protection, we tend to keep our beliefs so private that we rarely even acknowledge them to ourselves. There is however, a useful 3-step process which can hep you to uncover your beliefs about a subject. The approach is based on the landmark work of Otto Scharmer in his book *Theory-U*, in which he details how we can enact change both as individuals and as a society. Scharmer points out that before we can co-create a new and exciting future we must uncover our beliefs about our current situation and what we want to change. In order to achieve this he describes a definite 3-step process of inquiry which leads to the discovery of our deepest beliefs. The first step is to consider our thoughts, then our feelings and finally our beliefs. We use this progressive approach in our coaching work, and in the design of our training events for global corporations and it is highly effective.

Take five minutes now to write down what you think about your priority need on the hierarchy of needs. Nobody will see your answers, so you can be completely and brutally honest with yourself. There are no wrong or right answers to this question. Simply write down what you believe about security, love, esteem, achievement, or self-actualization – whichever is your priority need.

The initial level only scratch the surface of course and is more focused on the cognitive aspects. We tend to see shorter answers and often cliches responses to this question and that's a good start.

Now you can approach the second question. How does your priority need from the hierarchy of needs make you feel emotionally? E.g. Does it make you feel overwhelmed, sad, excited? Write the full list of emotions you feel about your priority need.

The final step is to write down your beliefs about your priority need. It can be useful to look at the list of emotions you wrote down in the last question and to ask yourself "What's the reason I feel [emotion] about this need?" What do you truly believe about your next level? This is the breakthrough question so spend as long as you need to write down your answers.

You should now feel that you have a much deeper understanding of yourself and what may be holding you back from achieving your priority need. The next step is to spend time each day challenging the negative beliefs that are holding you back. Challenge them with logic and replace them with balanced, realistic beliefs that encourage and energize you. You can't only think your way to success, it takes real action to achieve anything in life. For this reason, you must build in concrete steps that will give you the confidence that you can achieve your goal.

For example lets imagine that your priority need is security, and you answered that security is about having savings in the bank, living in a good neighborhood and that it makes you feel a little worried emotionally. Let's also imagine that the reason for this worry is that you don't believe that you can attain that level of security because of your current financial commitments and the belief that your salary will not increase in the current financial climate. Challenging that belief could include focusing on what you can do to make yourself more valuable in the jobs market, learning new and valuable skills, developing a valuable network at potential employers and exercising financial discipline daily. You may also be able to think of times when you have been in a difficult situation and came out the winner.

By focusing on challenging the limiting beliefs and taking action each day, we begin to build solid confidence in the belief that we can achieve our priority needs. This is the a very powerful way to make progress in your life and to feel energized. We use this approach extensively in our coaching and corporate training work and encourage you to master the skill too.

Motivation Hack 2 | Cognitive Consonance and Value – Goal – Action Alignment

How many times have you made a goal that you gave up on? How many times have you been given a goal that wasn't yours and it made you feel fatigued just thinking about it? No doubt you felt a surge of guilt and disappointment if the goal was not met. Have you ever felt that deep yet muffled feeling of anxiety from procrastinating around an important project?

It has been known and taught for thousands of years that we should live our lives true to our authentic selves. It is mentioned by the great philosophers and in many religious texts. The most famous sages of history elaborate that we should ensure that our daily actions are in alignment with our values, goals, and intentions. The concept has become more and more popular in recent years with value-based leadership, in particular becoming part of many corporate philosophies. Feeling properly aligned in our lives is a very powerful way to feel energized.

Nathaniel Branden, the godfather of self-esteem psychology (and philosophy), ascribed the alignment of values, intentions, and actions as one of the foundations of self-esteem, in addition to being honest with oneself. As we know, when we feel high self-esteem, we undoubtedly feel high energy and vitality at the same time.

In psychology, when our actions are at odds with our core beliefs and values, we experience a feeling of discomfort called "cognitive dissonance." The theory of cognitive dissonance was proposed by social psychologist Leon Festinger in 1957 and has not only endured time, but its neural basis has since been identified.

Festinger proposed that there are two possible states which relate to our thoughts and behaviors and how closely they are aligned. First, he described a consonant relationship in which our actions and our thoughts, beliefs, and intentions are aligned. For example, you may worry about your weight and plan to eat salad for dinner, and that evening you follow through on your plan and do indeed eat a salad. Kudos to you, for your beliefs, intentions, thoughts, and actions are aligned! This is cognitive consonance, and it is our optimal state. If, however, you are worried about your weight and plan to eat a salad for dinner but decide on a cheeseburger and a chocolate sundae instead, your beliefs, intentions, thoughts, and behaviors are not aligned, and you may well feel some guilt, anxiety, and discomfort as a result. This is Festinger's second state, called cognitive dissonance, and is at odds with a feeling of happiness, well-being, and vitality.

We experience that same feeling when we are faced with two difficult choices. The feeling is not always a pleasant one, which makes sense, as cognitive dissonance activates the same system in our brains that make us feel unhappy when we make mistakes.[144] Essentially, we don't like being wrong and we like our views, our beliefs, and actions to be well aligned. Suddenly the need for strong goals becomes compelling. With strong goals, we are more likely to be clear about our everyday decisions and to avoid cognitive dissonance.

It's when we *don't* have a clear goal or purpose that we begin to get into trouble, as competing options can create cognitive dissonance and that uneasy, slightly anxious feeling. Choices are confusing because our brains try to work out what's best as it scrambles to figure out our long-term, medium-term, and short-term objectives as they relate to the choices presented and the beliefs and values we hold. This is, of course, a huge load for the brain to process and it's all done in the energy-hungry prefrontal cortex (PFC). This means a lot more PFC action than would have been needed if we had chosen a clear goal. It also exposes us to the possibility of feeling guilt, disappointment, and all of the things that sap our energy and vitality. Who wouldn't be fatigued?!

Without goals, small obstacles become roadblocks, because all we can see and focus on is the obstacle. If, however, we know what we want and where we want to go in advance, if we have a goal, the problems become minor bumps in the road. The choices become more clear-cut. We experience less cognitive dissonance and more cognitive consonance. This makes us feel certain and energized.

Researchers from the Max Planck Institute in Leipzig, in collaboration with colleagues from St. Petersburg and Moscow Universities, shed some light on this phenomenon and looked more closely at an area of the brain called the posterior medial frontal cortex (pMFC). This area is associated with the behavior change we observe with cognitive dissonance. This is the same area of the brain that is associated with the reward prediction error we discussed earlier.

Researchers asked the test subjects to rate their preferences between different kinds of foods and snacks, from chocolate bars to vegetables. Once they had the preferences in order they showed two of the foods on a screen and asked the subjects to choose. The subjects were unaware that the scheming researchers only showed them choices that were above 6/10 on their personal preference scale so that they were likely to be shown chocolate and cookies on the same screen. Reaction time was used as an indicator of the level of cognitive dissonance. The researchers found that the PFC experienced a strong negative signal around 60ms after the choice was made, which is an indication of the discomfort we feel when we are faced with a tough choice and have to make a conflicted decision. Researchers also confirmed the theory that we adjust our preferences to suit our decision *after* it is made by downgrading our previous preferences. This is possibly to reduce the feeling of discomfort.

We have many curious methods of dealing with cognitive dissonance. We attempt to resolve the conflict through a mix of avoidance, self-justification, and devaluation of our pre-existing beliefs. Think about the jilted lover who replaces idealized devotion to his partner for a "didn't like her anyway" attitude, or the person who assures themselves that they're just big-boned after giving up on their 10th diet this year. In a sense, we align ourselves, but this post-justification is hardly the optimal way to do it and is in essence an inner conflict – not fertile ground for feeling energized and definitely fertile ground for burnout and fatigue.

The specific emotions that can arise from cognitive dissonance are shame, embarrassment, and guilt, which are sometimes referred to as the self-conscious emotions, with guilt being top of that list. Neurologically, many specific areas of the brain are involved in self-conscious emotions that lead to the feeling of cognitive dissonance. These areas are the fronto-temporo-limbic, the medial orbitofrontal gyrus, the medial frontal gyrus, the posterior cingulate gyrus, the anterior temporal lobe, the superior temporal sulcus (STS), and the subcortical structures, such as the amygdala and hypothalamus. Phew! That's a whole lot of brain to process emotions of guilt, shame, and embarrassment. It's no wonder we feel tired when faced with difficult choices, or worse, when our actions and goals aren't aligned.

Psychologist Roy Baumeister from Florida State University theorized that guilt, in particular, has a social function which prevents us from doing things that would jeopardize a relationship's harmony, such as cheating and stealing. He theorized that it "motivates people to treat partners well and avoid transgressions, minimizing inequities and enabling less powerful partners to get their way, and redistributing emotional distress." [145]

Baumeister is essentially alluding to the idea that humans need to follow a set of social rules that guarantee our survival as a species, a very peaceful harmonious state and fertile ground for energy and vitality. This can be easily explained with the example of music. Musical consonance and dissonance is the difference between sounding in tune (consonance) and sounding like a 2-year-old hitting the wrong keys in a scale (dissonance). It's a great metaphor for the cognitive dissonance we feel in our lives when we are not aligned. But, being aligned could be just part of the story – after all, aren't we aligned just to our most important next task? This doesn't seem to be the complete answer to that "gnawing" guilty feeling that even those with the utmost integrity feel from time to time.

In an experiment, researchers looked deeper into the possible reasons for consonance and dissonance in music and the reasons that dissonance feels so awful and consonance feels so pleasant. They took musically untrained students and ran a series of experiments aimed at teaching participants simple music rules. Some were taught basic musical rules using dissonant scales (i.e., discordant-sounding ones) and others were taught using consonant ones (i.e., harmonious-sounding ones). The results showed that participants were able to learn and apply the rules using a consonant scale as an *anchor* from which to spot the errors in the test.[146] They hypothesized that having a consonant set of rules from which the brain can map its environment musically may extend outside of the musical realm to areas including statistics and linguistics.

Adherence to a "set of rules" provides a feeling of pleasantness. We know that commitment to life rules, principles, and beliefs are as fundamental to the emotional sense of energy and vitality as diet and sleep are to the physiological side of the equation. Those life rules should serve as the "true north," from which an energizing and exciting vision and goals can be derived for the highest levels of energy and vitality.

Take the time now to write down the unwritten rules you live your life by. Be completely honest with yourself, you don't have to share them with anyone. Your rules are most likely tied to the values you hold dear. Again, you may not like the some of rules you see when they are written in front of you, but there is a next step to this exercise.

The rules you wrote down are your unofficial guidelines in life, but always remember that they are just that – guidelines – and as none has or will ever have complete wisdom to know everything knowable, be prepared to challenge and update them regularly. Remember that sometimes our rules can be too rigid and can end up hurting our interests (and other people), but at least knowing what rules you've been living by is a great way to realign either the rules or the goals you have, in order to stay in cognitive consonance.

So, in conclusion, cognitive consonance with our priority need from the hierarchy of needs, and alignment with a set of life principles is a powerful energy hack. Decisions become easier and your brain knows that it's investing its energy wisely. The vitality of feeling motivated is the surefire sign that you're on the right track. Merely acting to avoid problems isn't really the kind of positive vitality that we are looking for. If we are serious about our journey to vitality, then we need to be aligned with ourselves.

Motivation Hack 3 | Positive Psychology

Positive psychology is the study of what is 'right' with people rather than what's 'wrong' with them. It grew largely from the recognition of an imbalance in clinical psychology, in which most research focuses on mental illness. Personal health and wellness goes beyond the absence of major mental illnesses or psychological disorders. Martin Seligman, leading authority in positive psychology, at the start of his career discovered the power of optimism. He argued that optimism precedes success rather than the other way around. By implementing an aptitude test to screen optimism, he was able to increase sales of optimistic agents at Metlife Insurance by a staggering 56% compared to pessimistic sales representatives. Seligman's message was to enjoy a life of happiness that he proposed rested on 3 pillars; joy, engagement, and meaning. Meaning and values do, of course, go hand in hand as they relate to a transcendence beyond ourselves and towards a greater good, focused on a social perspective rather than on "me".

Social energy is defined as a generally motivated, engaged and active state generated by participating in something that one likes with another person, who independently shares the same feelings about the task or subject. Research demonstrates that people who find themselves as part of a group who experience social energy, score higher measures of attention, participation, connection, belonging, satisfaction, and absorption. Think about a sports crowd cheering for the same team, a mass of fans supporting an artist at a concert or the energy you get from a choir when they harmonize together in song. The social aspect of life is important for vitality, and, as we will see later, has a neural basis.

Crucially, Seligman suggested that living a life in line with six core values is associated with feeling energized as opposed to fatigued.

Core Strength	Components
1. **Wisdom and knowledge**: cognitive strengths that entail the acquisition of knowledge.	Creativity; curiosity; judgment and open-mindedness; love of learning; perspective.
2. **Courage**: emotional strengths that involve the exercise of will to accomplish goals in the face of opposition, external or internal.	Bravery; perseverance; honesty; zest.
3. **Humanity**: interpersonal strengths that involve tending and befriending.	Capacity to love and be loved; kindness; social intelligence.
4. **Justice**: civic strengths that underlie healthy community life.	Teamwork; fairness; leadership.
5. **Temperance**: strengths that protect against excess.	Forgiveness and mercy; modesty; prudence; self-regulation.
6. **Transcendence**: strengths that forge connections to the larger universe and provide meaning.	Appreciation of beauty and excellence; gratitude; hope; humor; religiousness and spirituality.

Seligman and others posit that living a life in line with these core values, which they describe as "core strengths of human goodness," helps us to feel positive emotions and subsequently feel energized. This is completely in line with our own experience with our coaching clients and within organizations. Seligman should know; the list is the result of a large and significant research project spanning many cultures across the globe.

For energy, the benefits of positive psychology stretch beyond the positive values and traits of Seligman's list. Barbara Frederickson's "broaden and build" theory of positive emotions suggests that positive emotions increase people's attention, expand cognition (e.g., curiosity and creativity) and behaviors (e.g., exploration and play), and consequently foster physical, intellectual, and social resources (e.g., intelligence, mastery, and social competence) for optimal functioning. Frederickson's theory defines the very traits that we associate with living lives that are high in vitality and energy. So, how to hack it? What can we do in our daily lives and routines to enjoy the benefits of positive psychology?

One way is to spend time to consider the positive things that happened to you each day. The number is not important; it's the process of scanning your day for positives, as opposed to scanning your day for negatives. Positively re-framing situations in a more balanced way, as opposed to just disasters, is central to positive psychology. One person's disaster is another's learning opportunity – or maybe just not as bad as you first thought. Indeed, the high energy of the successful entrepreneurs that sparked our interest in this subject may well be derived from this source.

In his book *Entrepreneurship for the Rest of Us*, journalist and author Paul Brown explored the traits of the most successful entrepreneurs in the U.S. The results were surprising and his point was emphatically made: entrepreneurs view failure as a "gift." His observation, from hundreds of interviews over many years, was that entrepreneurs simply take small steps, learn from failures, and then build on what they discover and repeat the cycle until they win. It is what Brown describes in his book as the "entrepreneurs' secret."

Clearly the "entrepreneurs' secret" is the trait of people who can re-frame failures as the positive learning experiences we associate with positive psychology, which is another clue that practicing positive psychology is a great hack for feeling positive energy and vitality.

Positive Psychology is founded on Seligman's belief that "people want to lead meaningful and fulfilling lives, to cultivate what is best within themselves, and to enhance their experiences of love, work, and play". The pursuit of happiness has been a common quest in most civilizations throughout the centuries. We have never met a person whose meaning of life didn't involve happiness to some extent. From being happy themselves to making others happy, happiness is always an underlying intention.

The truth is that happiness is not just a plastered smile, it is not a specific emotion, but a global state. We all have an emotional base level. This base is susceptible to peaks and troughs, but the base changes very slowly and is usually quite constant. The baseline is what we call happiness, the positive peaks are joys and the troughs are sorrows.[147] For example, when a person gets a pay raise they are usually happy, motivation is at a peak and we feel like we have all the energy in the world and can achieve anything we desire. As time passes by, the person gets used to their new salary, the initial euphoria diminishes and their emotional level returns to the initial baseline level of happiness. However, these moments, happy or sad, gradually influence the baseline.[148] Although we do not have full control over what happens in our lives, we do have control over how they affect us. Likewise, we have control over different factors that influence our happiness. Just like energy itself, happiness is basically controlled by two dimensions, internal factors and external factors, or what scientists call endogenous and exogenous factors respectively. The external factors are the things in our environment that stimulate a response such as a beautiful view, an angry boss or, as we will see, the weather.

The internal factors are those dictated by biology, cognition and personality. Biological influences are a compound of our temperament, genetics, neurotransmitter balances, endocrine factors, hormones, and physical and mental state. Science points out that this dimension is responsible for 35% -50% of happiness.[149] While there is no gene for happiness, genetics does orchestrate the chemical composition behind mood and emotional processing.

There are a many ways to approach each event that happens in our lives. No matter what the situation is, there is always a perspective that is, even marginally, more positive. The best way to protect your energy and vitality each day is to practice gratitude and to seek out the positive collateral of any situation.[150] Several scientific studies show that grateful people experience more positive emotions throughout the day, have a much greater sense of belonging and have significantly lower rates of depression and stress.[151] Rather than getting mad by assuming that the terrible driver who just cut in on you is a genuinely nasty person, try instead to imagine that perhaps it's a hard working mother who's running late to pick her daughter, or maybe even acing to help a grandparent who called for help in an emergency.

Daily deliberate practice of this skill, which is very fun to do, gradually changes our behavior and thinking patterns. Whilst we should to be realistic that not everything in life is idyllic, there is always a way to approach events in a more positive light, even if its simply acknowledging that things could be worse. By doing this, we reserve our energy for things that really matter to us, and we avoid giving into anger, which saps our energy and leads to burnout.

Empathy is an essential human characteristic that allows us to share and understand the internal states of others, their beliefs and intentions. In fact, the scientific community has found that our emotional states are highly influenced by the people in our presence.[152] So much so that when a person in an MRI sees positive images, they interpret them as far more positive if a friend is present compared to seeing the same image alone.[153] Even further, it has been proven that the emotions of those around us are contagious. Several replications of the same scientific study show that the mere presence of happy people increases the happiness of others around them significantly.[154] This also applies to energy. Social energy is also greatly studied in positive psychology. You have probably experienced social energy when you are at a sports game, a music concert, or when you step into a bar with a good vibe. Exposure to social energy is always a great way to boost our vitality levels.[155]

People who volunteer and care for others have significantly lower rates of depression and significantly higher happiness and vitality rates.[156] Although volunteering is often collaborating in an organization or club, it can also be as simple as contacting an acquaintance or friend that we know is alone or is going through a tough time. Being aware of others not only reminds us of all the reasons why we should be grateful, but it gives us a feeling of responsibility and achievement too.

When we help others and see the positive effect we have generated, our body secretes serotonin.[157] This feeling of achievement and satisfaction reinforces altruistic behavior and strengthens our chances of being happy. Helping others also reinforces the idea that we are useful, that we have a reason for being, that we are valuable, that we have something we can give, that there are lives we can change and the feeling that our energy and time are well spent.

Giving a sense and meaning to our actions and behaviors highly affect our happiness levels and therefor our energy. When we have a good reason to wake up each morning, when we have a real purpose to take action, or when there is a worthwhile reason to fight, it is much easier to feel vitalized. Communication and introspection are a key here. In one study, researchers confirmed that writing or talking with others regularly about our experiences, contributes to our happiness and well-being.[158] Communicating our thoughts, feelings and emotions often has a sanitizing effect. The explanation goes far beyond mere venting. When we make tangible, either by speaking or writing our most intimate thoughts, we create a situation in which we are invited to reflect on what has happened, as it has happened, why it has happened and what we can do about it. It also helps us to take a step backwards and to see the situation in a more general way, disconnecting and observing our lives almost in the third person.

There is no single rule or recipe that applies to everyone to guarantee a happy and energized life. There is no pill to guarantees that life will be perfect life. It may sometimes seem that another person has it easier to be happier than you, but remember that there is someone else who thinks the same of you too. "If I had that, if I were like that, then I would be happy". But the truth is that we all have something to be happy about, and something to bring us sorrow too.

It is important to remember again that in human psychology our perspective of happiness is not objective. In a study, a group of participants were given the choice between a cup or a quantity of money. They were asked how much money it would take for them to choose the money over the cup, which indicated it's perceived value in the situation. The average amount was $3.50. Another group of participants was given a cup and asked how much money they would have to get in exchange for their cup. The average this time was $7.12. In both circumstances the cup was the same, but the fact of owning it, made this object twice as valuable.[159]

Several studies that have followed lottery winners show that winning large sums of money gives great joy. Nonetheless, it only takes a couple of months for these lucky winners to return to their baseline level of happiness, the one they had before the big win.[160]

What is your motivation? What makes you happy? By making sure you have a positive outlook of life you can assure higher levels of vitality and energy and avoid fatigue and burnout.

Take the time now to write down a list of all the things that make you feel happy, no matter how big or small. It could include taking a walk in nature, sleeping in for a while, seeing the smile on your partners face, or laughing with an old friend. Write down what's true for you.

Add to the list all of the things in your life that you are grateful for. You could include the money you have in the bank, no matter how little, gratitude for the roof over your head that keeps you safe, for the loving relationships in your life or simply for being alive.

Keep the list visible each day and look at it often. Update the list as you discover more and more ways to enjoy positive emotions and happiness.

Let the list be a guide that steers you towards the activities and situations that bring you happiness and enjoy the energy and vitality that happiness brings.

Motivation Hack 4 | Locus of Control

Being efficient with our hard earned energy is vitally important, yet it's surprisingly easy to waste our energy, especially on the things that we cannot control. One of the most important aspects of energy efficiency is what's known in psychology as the "locus of control."

People with a so-called *internal* locus of control focus on the things in their life that they *can* control and they worry less about the things they *can't* control. Conversely, people with an *external* locus of control worry disproportionately about the things that are *outside* of their control, including what others think. A person with an external locus of control will spend more energy worrying about possible consequences to themselves and their families rather than on the things that are within their control. A person with an internal locus of control will immediate think about the things they can do to influence or control the situation for the best outcome. Psychologists attribute an internal locus of control to positive outcomes, and it is a central part of positive psychology – which makes it good for our energy and vitality too.

Wasting your mental energy on things outside of your locus of control can have damaging effects to your decisions long after the event. Some evidence from an experiment at the University of Duisburg-Essen, in which a group of people were asked to solve anagrams, some solvable and some unsolvable, illustrates this very clearly. [161]

Following the anagram test, participants were asked to complete another test to determine their decision-making performance. Surprisingly, the subjects who wasted their time on the unsolvable anagrams made worse decisions than those who were given the solvable anagrams.

The researchers concluded that feelings of what's called *learned helplessness* had been a major factor. Learned helplessness, is the state in which a person feels that they are powerless in a situation, even when a solution exists. This pessimistic state is an enemy of energy, vitality and the all-important internal locus of control. It's worth noting that the feeling of being in an uncontrollable situation induces cognitive performance similar to that of patients who suffer depression.[162]

The salient point here is not to waste our precious energy pushing against doors that will not open, but to focus our energy on the things that we really can tangibly influence.

Let's do an exercise together. Take a piece of paper right now. Write down a list of things that are concerning you right now and the reasons that each is causing you concern; e.g., "My partner and I are arguing. The reason this concerns me is that he/she may leave me and I will be lonely."

1. Write down the things that are outside your circle of control. In this instance it could be, "I cannot force my partner to be happy or calm. This is outside of my locus of control."

2. Now write down the things that you can change. "I can focus on being calm myself;" "I can write down the points that he/she made as if they were said without anger;" "I can honestly appraise whether or not they were right;" "I can express that I have understood what they said and this is what I will do in response;" or, "this is all I can do, without relying on any expectation on their part."

3. Do this for each area of your life and add any relevant actions to your to-do list.

By taking this action, you will have focused your energy on your internal locus of control and you will be following a principle of positive psychology. By being efficient with your energy, you will have a lot more energy left for the other aspects of your life.

Motivation Hack 5 | Visualization

Have you ever held a goal that you thought was simply unattainable? You probably struggled to commit your energy to the goal because your mind simply didn't believe that it was realistic. Our efficient minds are not easily convinced to trade their precious resources once the adrenaline rush of starting a new project has subsided. So many goals lie in the graveyard of noble plans, starved of belief. If this has ever happened to you, visualization is the skill to master.

Visualization is a staple of sports psychology. Athletes, often guided by a psychologist, imagine a sporting scene such as a big game or performance. The athlete then imagines that they are in the game, visualizing the sights, sounds, emotions, and even the tactile feel of the moment. The visualizations typically involve not only perfect performances, but also pressure situations like being behind in a game or experiencing stage fright. The athlete or performer then visualizes a winning response to the pressure.

Eight-time Ukrainian gymnastics champion and Olympian Nadezhda Belavtseva confided to us that gymnasts often use visualization techniques when recovering from injury.

"Before going to the competition site, the gymnast can several times undergo an exercise in the head, and all her body is in tension. All the movements that she repeats in her head, impulses of the brain, go into action. Very many athletes during the recovery from surgery or a long rest are engaged in a few minutes of playing in the mind of the training process."

Belavtseva, one of the most talented athletes we have ever come across, describes a unique method of visualization which involves both tension of the muscles and visualization for powerful results. Researchers believe that muscles, in response to the visualization, are actually engaged and activated to some extent. So, with visualization, can we convince our mind that what it perceives as impossible is actually possible?

When legendary golfer Jack Nicklaus famously talked about "going to the movies," he was describing the way he visualized each shot before swinging the golf club in competition. He knew that if he had visualized the shot well, his body would respond and when he stood over the ball that very shot would materialize.

At the Beijing Olympics in 2006, Olympian and swimming giant Michael Phelps showed us the true power of visualization. A literal giant in Phelps' case, the swimmer visualized multiple scenarios which paid off big time in the 200m men's butterfly final. Phelps's goggles filled with water as soon as he entered the water, but he kept calm, counted his strokes, and powered to the finish to take the gold medal with a world-record time. Phelps revealed in an interview with the Washington Post, that he had visualized every possible scenario beforehand, including the eventuality that his "suit ripped or goggles broke." His mind believed that it could deal with any eventuality and this in turn breeds gold medal winning confidence. A wardrobe malfunction in the pool? No problem; he'd already visualized his response. For you too, visualizing how you will respond positively in a situation that may be causing you some anxiety, will help you to prepare you body and mind to win. This is the perfect antidote to leaned helplessness and the inevitable feelings of anxiety and fatigue we often when faced with a mountain to climb.

So, who visualized visualization? In 1971 at the University of Western Ontario, psychologist Allan Paivio proposed the "dual-coding theory of learning" in which he postulated that we learn using verbal associations and mental imagery in a process known as dual-coding. The idea of dual-coding has endured and been confirmed with experiments in neuroscience. Later, in 1985, Paivio took his idea further and created a framework for visualization in sports which has been predominant ever since. He proposed that there are cognitive and motivational aspects to imagery that can affect actual behavior. The cognitive aspects include strategy and specific skill rehearsal whilst the motivational aspects are focused on winning, controlling emotions, and overcoming challenging and unforeseen situations – in essence, creating the belief and confidence to succeed.[163]

In both sports and music, professionals with higher skill levels utilize visualization more than their less-skilled counterparts. Further, the ability to visualize is not a skill that everyone possesses, and researchers found that those that use it the most in sports tend to possess a greater ability for it, which is logical.

In their review of the available research on imagery, scholars from the University of London Music School noted that, "Simply asking musicians to engage in imagery is not enough. Imagery is a skill, it can be practiced, and improvements may be made over time, resulting in enhanced effectiveness of the imagery. Thus, by encouraging musicians to practice imagery and teaching them when and what to image at appropriate times, their imagery may become more effective, and ideally they will experience the corresponding benefits of the effective use of imagery." [176]

The researchers suggested a two-step model for visualization to maximize its effectiveness:

First, decide the situation. Is it a rehearsal or is it "lights, camera, action" time, i.e. the big performance?

Second, decide whether you want to visualize technique (e.g., playing the notes of a song) or one of the motivational aspects, such as the feeling of a winning performance or coming back from 3-0 down to beat your opponents in the second half of the game.

The aim of the exercise is better focus, technique, and confidence in your visualization skills. Researchers note that the key aspects to make a successful visualization are firstly, your ability to generate images, and secondly, the methods you use to create a real experience. The goal is to convince the mind that it is real, making it believe that you have enjoyed a positive and real experience, creating a vivid memory in the process. The full sequence is detialed on the opposite page.

It's time to practice. Take five minutes to follow the sequence of steps detailed below. It's okay to get it wrong – it's just practice. Over time, you will become a master.

Try it now, and repeat the exercise as often as you can to reinforce the belief that you *can* achieve your goal.

You may have found the experience awkward. The mind wanders, and it's often hard to maintain focus. It's helpful to see each visualization as practice. You may even find it useful to go online to find a guided imagery coach to help you.

We believe that visualization is an excellent hack for vitality because it helps you to create belief and confidence in achieving a goal you may otherwise have found daunting. Remember that "success orbits around confidence," and confidence comes in part from the realistic belief that you can overcome your challenges. When we lose confidence and belief, we can feel defeated, fatigued and burned-out. When you feel low on belief, visualization is a powerful way to get it back, restoring your energy and vitality in the process. It takes practice, but the rewards are worth the effort.

Step 1
Choose a goal: perhaps the next Maslow level, a task, or a new belief that you want to visualize. The function is motivation. The situation will be experiencing yourself successfully achieving the goal.

Step 2
Choose your Anchor: Remember a time that you achieved something worthwhile. What was it and where were you? This will be your anchor. You will first recall this scene and experience the great emotions associated with it.

Step 3
When you're ready, focus on breathing in through your nose and count each breath to ten, one at a time. Notice the breath when you exhale. The purpose is to clear your thoughts.

Step 4
Recall the anchor scene. Think about the scene in as much detail as you can: where you were, what you could see, the moment of celebration, the "winning" feeling, and how good you felt.

Step 5
Now, holding onto that winning feeling, imagine the future goal. Imagine achieving the goal in as much detail as possible. Where will you be and what can you see? Imagine celebrating, and take as much time as you can to experience and enjoy that winning feeling once again.

Step 6
Open your eyes, take a big stretch, and congratulate yourself once more for taking the time to visualize success.

Summary

Each of the many hacks in this section are links that, when used together, form a powerful chain strong enough to lift you to a new level of energy and vitality. We've called this process the "motivation chain." (see next page)

The motivation chain enables you to leverage the nature of your brain in order to harness the energizing power of motivation. The chain involves committing energy only to activities which are in line with your highest priority needs and within your locus of control. This highly aligned sequence is designed to increase cognitive consonance which in turn delivers the energizing feelings of confidence, certainty and self belief.

Motivation Chain

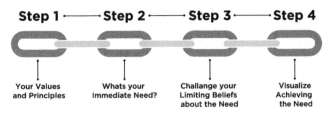

We have listed the links of the motivation chain for you to follow below and we encourage you to practice as you read through the steps.

Values and Principles
- Which three positive values truly define who you are as a person (e.g., winning, achievement, intellection, self-actualization, family, loyalty, fun, etc.)?

- Write down the unofficial rules you live your life by, and update them as needed to serve you well for the future.

Immediate Goals | Ensuring Cognitive Consonance
- Where are you currently on Maslow's hierarchy of needs: Survival, love and belonging, esteem, achievement or self-actualization?
- What is your next unmet level on the hierarchy? This is your immediate priority need (e.g., security).
- Add some detail and define exactly what you need. For example, if your priority need is security, what type of security (e.g. physical, emotional, financial etc.)

Plan
- Write down five things you need to do in order to achieve your immediate goal (e.g., updating your resume).
- Using Pareto's principal (aka the 80/20 rule), one of the items on the list will give you the biggest impact. Which one is it?

Beliefs
- Write down your beliefs about the immediate need. What do you think about it, how does it make you feel, and finally what do you believe about it deep down?
- Ask yourself, "What's the reason I believe this?"
- Challenge the beliefs and develop more rational beliefs about the priority need.

Visualize
- Close your eyes and recall a time when you achieved something challenging and felt great. Where were you? Access that memory and relive the winning feeling.

- Now, create a vivid picture in your mind of satisfying the immediate need. What can you see and hear?
- Finish by visualizing as vividly as possible the experience of having that winning feeling once again in your future scene.

As we have discovered, energy and self-motivation go hand in hand. To feel energized, we need to focus on the things that are important to us, both because they represent who we are authentically and also because they really are our top priority and most pressing need.

The value of perspective cannot be overstated for managing energy. Perspective has the capability to make a molehill out of a mountain, reduce stress, and make goals and objectives feel more achievable. It's the difference between waking up bewildered and terrified as a small piece on a board game surrounded by fierce-looking wooden figures, and being the grandmaster chess player of that very game, experienced with the rules and tactics, in control of the game, and clear on your next moves. Knowing your goals and values, having an internal locus of control, and being aware of your next immediate motivational need, provides that perspective.

If you are determined enough to work up through each of the levels in Maslow's hierarchy of needs, eventually reaching the level of self-actualization, you will have achieve the immense satisfaction of achieving everything you can with the gifts that you have, This is where vitality and energy truly reside, and it is the level that we associate with the greatest entrepreneurs and most energized people on the planet.

ENERGY EFFICIENCY AND ENVIRONMENT

If having more energy is our goal, being efficient with the energy that we do have is transformational. Imagine a state of living where all of your energy is invested into the things that you truly love and to the stuff that really matters. An emotional state where energy becomes vitality and productivity becomes limitless.

It is also import to remember that as humans we respond to the environment in which we live, moment-to-moment. From the room that you are in, to the people that surround you, to the rain or shine of the day's weather, how we feel emotionally is a direct response to these factors. Our environment can be inspiring and it can be distracting, it can invigorate us or it can drain us. We cannot master our energy, vitality and beat fatigue without the skills to master our environment, and reaction to it too.

In this chapter we will show you how to master the distracting elements of your environment and how to focus your energy with great efficiency on the stuff that really matters, all according to science and a little wisdom from the ancients.

Concentration, Flow and Mindfulness

Ever been so absorbed in a book that you lost track of time? Ever been so ensconced by an activity that you simply don't want to go to bed? Maybe you worked for a long, uninterrupted period, deeply engaged with energy and vitality, and didn't even feel tired when you finished. Welcome to the "flow state."

The flow state is a state of deeply engaged immersion into an activity. As alluded to above, you may sometimes experience flow as a sense of being lost in a book, as the background sounds fade to silent and you become focused on each emerging word on the page. This state of flow is highly productive, and with a little knowledge, we can access it in our workplace and in our private activities. It helps us to have deeply significant and rewarding experiences with minimal energy and maximal enjoyment. However, in our constantly interrupted lives, flow is somewhat rare. Instant messenger and beeping apps pervade our consciousness, vying for our attention like 4-year-olds at Disney World.

The mental state we are really describing when we talk about an energy-efficient deep connection would be more appropriately known as "immersion." The word seems fitting, as immersion into water conjures up the image of disconnecting with our normal, more familiar environment and submerging into a different world. Your senses and cognition are heightened for the specific activity of being underwater; you are completely connected, focused and totally committed, conscious of nothing else outside of the experience.

Playing chess may represent the closest opportunity to the state of immersion than any other. Let's return to the fascinating experiment with the chess players we looked at earlier. One observation of the researchers was the way in which advanced players versus the novice players utilized their cognitive attention. What exactly were they focusing on?

Researchers noted that during a chess game, novice players had a tendency to visually scan the chessboard, taking in irrelevant information and wasting their mental resources as well as valuable time. The advanced players, on the other hand, focused immediately on the critical aspects of the game, ignoring the irrelevant bits, which left them more time and mental resources to evaluate the winning move.[164] They were immersed cognitively in the key aspects of the game and had inhibited the distraction of the irrelevant aspects. This is the key to immersion.

Cognitively, the players were working through the many iterations and consequences of moves and countermoves so the prefrontal cortex (PFC) would still be highly active but operating with efficiency and coming closer to its full potential. This immersion and focus on the cognitive aspects of the game is subtly different to the "zone," often referred to by elite sportsmen and women, in which, it is reported, cognition is inhibited and senses are heightened. The grand master chess players focus attention solely on the cognitive aspects, the elite sportsmen focus solely on the sensory aspects similar to the state of mindfulness.

Mindfulness and vitality go together like dancers in a flamenco. Mindfulness allows our mind to be free of the cerebral clutter that distracts us from experiencing every moment. How can we truly experience vitality if we can't even experience reality? As Bob Marley said, "Some people feel the rain, other people just get wet." Experiencing life in a mindful way is at the very essence of enjoying life, yet a look around any café, restaurant, or even dinner table is a tragic reminder of how distracted we have become from reality. Eating time is now a time to catch up on email, or to cram in a few more minutes of work, or just zone out into a pseudo-reality where we observe other people's lives through our magical rectangular glowing windows i.e. your phone.

Mindful eating offers a great way to get your mindfulness time during the day as part of your routine. We discovered the Japanese tradition of eating mindfully with all five senses: it is called *Gokan de Ajiwau*.

Gokan De Ajiwau means taking a few seconds to observe the taste and other sensations of eating.

Eating with all five senses (=五感 *gokan* in Japanese) is something people in Japan do effortlessly as a second nature. It's a great food culture that appreciates the subtlety of flavors. Food-related TV shows are always featuring their presenters eating unique foods from around Japan, but what's striking is that there is always a focus on the senses' reaction to the food, from extreme close-ups of the visual appearance, to the presenter communicating their delight at the taste, texture, and smell of the food. In Japanese movies and TV dramas as well, the sound of chewing is often enhanced. The five senses are: sight, smell, sound, texture, taste.

Mindfully observing the flavor and texture of food, and then savoring the flavor for a few seconds after swallowing, is a joy. Doing this alone develops mindfulness, as you are essentially observing a perception. This is a very powerful skill. You may be shocked at how oblivious you have been to the taste of the food you have been consuming for years. Like us, you may feel that you have regained consciousness after being in a culinary coma of sorts. We believe that enjoying even the simplest things, such as the taste and texture of your food, moment by moment, is by far the best way to enjoy vitality.

How Distraction Saps your Energy

You may not be aware of it, but you can always hear the sound of your refrigerator when you are in your home (assuming you don't live in a sprawling palace). Try turning it off and see how strange the room sounds. Our brains receive sound, and that sound is processed at the rostrum brainstem sitting at the bottom of the brain. The rostrum brainstem is controlled by the prefrontal cortex (PFC); the PFC tells it what to focus on, and it then tries its best to filter out as much of the irrelevant noise as possible.[165] It's another fascinating example of the way that the brain is always "on" at a very high level, even if it just to inhibit an incoming signal.

Interference is all around us, pervasively corroding away our ability to focus. Whether we are interrupted by a new project, an unexpected visit from the boss, a thought about a loved one, or the sound of a bird outside the window, we are interrupted nonetheless.

As we saw earlier, our brains are always operating at a very high baseline of energy usage. Conscious thought or activation actually accounts for very little extra expenditure of energy.[166]

So, while it may seem quiet in the brain in terms of attention and cognition, a lot is actually going on, and that includes processing the visual and auditory chatter subconsciously. Researchers from Yale University have shown a whopping 80% of the energy use in the brain is used for what's called "glutamate cycling," which happens when there is active signaling in the brain.[167] In fact, research shows that the brain uses a lot of energy all of the time, in a balance of excitation and inhibition of neurons. The neurons are always active in either of these two states; both use energy. Given the huge energy requirements of the brain, this means that the brain is doing a lot of processing *all* of the time, and that includes processing distractions. We do, however, have a very limited capacity for attention.

As a species, we evolved in more natural and hostile environments than our densely packed but relatively safe urban habitats. Saber-toothed tigers once lurked in the tall grass with other man-eating predators, making heightened senses essential for survival. In more recent times, our senses are kept equally occupied. Silence in any urban space is as extinct as the saber-toothed tiger, and in our malls and civic centers we are literally bombarded with signals screaming for our attention. We have never been allowed to relax as a species; we have lost, or maybe never had, the ability to focus – and it's not just environmental factors at play.

Here's a delightful challenge for you and, with practice, a hack that will help you to focus your attention and energy which involves eating with all five senses as we discussed in the last section. The next time that you drink a cup of coffee or tea, take the time to drink it mindfully. Savor the look, the taste, how the liquid feels in your mouth, and how it feels to swallow it, and put all of your attention to enjoying and noticing the taste that lingers on your tongue. You will be surprised by the detail that your mind can pick up when it really focuses on something. You may also be surprised how difficult the exercise is and, for some, you may be surprised by how little else you noticed in what was going on around you at the moment. So why was the task so difficult?

Our minds have only limited attentional resources. When we sit in Starbucks sipping our latte, it's unlikely that any of us pay the amount of attention just described in our mindful drinking challenge. Our minds would be simultaneously drawn to the people around us with minimal amounts of attentional resources paid to any specific distraction (generally speaking). Mindfully eating and drinking is one of our favorite hacks which we encourage you to do daily.

Unlike how our eyelids can block out our sight, it's not possible, without putting our hands over our ears, to block out ambient sounds. It's surprising, then, that when we arrive home at night after a hard day's work, that we can't hear the sound of the refrigerator, despite the fact that the sound waves are hitting our ears. It's the same for people who live next to a train line or busy road: after a while, we become accustomed to the sound and stop hearing it in our conscious mind.

As we mentioned at the introduction to this section of the book, at some level, our brain is using its resources to filter out what's not important from what is. This is often referred to as the "cocktail party effect." Coined by Colin Cherry in 1953, the phenomenon relates to our ability to selectively filter information that's useful to us, in this case, our name, being spoken across the room at a busy cocktail party. Somehow, we hear our name above the din of the soirée. Although this is likely due to the importance we place on our name since birth, it also relates to a wider range of auditory information that randomly occupies our soundscape each moment.

So why does this happen and why is this a possible energy hack? There are two models for auditory selectivity: the early processing method and the late processing method. Scientists are divided as to which is wrong or right, but there is without doubt a level of processing that we do subconsciously.

A sound signal enters the brain via the ear (clearly) and then through the auditory nerve to the auditory cortex. From there, it moves to the "Wernicke's area" in the left hemisphere. Sound that is deemed to be of importance will enter our working memory, which is located at our PFC and parietal areas. However, a logical connection with our long-term memory, i.e., a determination of the sound being relevant, must also occur.

With regards to the "own name recognition" we associate with the cocktail party phenomenon, researchers from the University of California San Diego and University of Nagoya revealed, using fMRI, that when not actively listening, the midbrain reticular formation, thalamus, insula, auditory cortex, and precuneus are indeed active nevertheless. In short, a network of brain regions, including the rostrum brainstem, is actively monitoring sounds for stuff that could be of importance to us, saving attentional resources but using energy too.

Evidence suggests that when it comes to vision, our brains primarily tunes into how the object moves – which would fit with the hunter hypothesis. In low light, for example, it may be hard to see whether a dark figure is a man-eating tiger or something more benign. Seeing the slow, stalking movement would be a dead giveaway.

Interestingly, the stuff that's happening in our peripheral vision isn't as big a problem. Research published in the brilliantly titled *Perception & Psychophysics*, and carried out by the Dutch Institute for Road Safety Research, showed that our attention is only interrupted by things that happen within our direct field of vision, the so-called "zoom lens theory."[168]

Try it for yourself right now. Take a look at the things in the space around you that are moving – maybe a tree outside the window with its branches and leaves swaying in the wind. Now look back to this page and, focusing on the words on it, see if you can still notice the movement. You should not be able to pick up any subtle movement at all.

There is a caveat. If we are already primed to expect important visual cues, our peripheral vision, or more accurately our peripheral attention, will indeed pick it up.[169] Thus, if we are expecting someone to walk into the room, our peripheral vision will pick it up as soon as it happens. This is a notably important ability for airline pilots, for whom blinking lights are vital signals.

Sound is a much bigger distraction than what happens in our peripheral field of vision, although we must admit that we struggle to focus on the page we are writing with the TV on in front of us and the sound muted. Researchers have become more and more aware of the effect of background noise on cognitive processing, especially with regards to working memory. Background noise has been found to be detrimental to learning and cognition. As trainers, we can vouch that ambient noise is highly distracting to learning, which requires focused and unbroken concentration, certainly in a classroom setting. [170]

So, both sight and sound are distracting; how about touch?

Touch is another way in which our brains exhibit an inhibiting action in order to allow focus on a specific stimulus. What do we mean by this? Touch involves a process known as lateral inhibition. When we experience touch in a specific area – the middle of our palm, for example – the nerve signals in the areas just around the contact area are inhibited. This creates a contrast and enables us to locate exactly where we are being touched. Try an experiment now. Blow gently onto the tip your middle finger and focus on the feeling. Now press the area just below the tip of your finger with a finger-nail and continue to blow. You can feel the sensation in the middle of the finger slightly reduce. This is an example of lateral inhibition and potentially a great painkiller! A complete digression, but interesting nonetheless.

So, what are our hacks for avoiding distraction in your environment, or what scientists call interference resolution?

Efficiency Hack 1 | Pink Noise or Earplugs

Clearly, wearing olive green ear defenders made for the flight deck of an aircraft carrier or a yellow pair meant for a construction site won't cut it in public. Cutting out sound is hard to do. Sound travels in air, so any gaps that are left between the ear canal and the outside world will leak sound. More than that, some sound waves of specific lengths are able to penetrate reasonably dense materials. Bass in particular, with its sound wave measured in meters, can easily penetrate the thin material of a foam earplug. Higher frequency sounds, with its more tightly packed soundwaves, are easier to stop, yet at the volumes played in restaurants and cafés, foam ear plugs are all but useless. The ubiquitous trumpet of a Starbucks soundtrack seems to be a sound wave all of its own, because no matter what method of ear defending we try, the trumpet always wins.

There are however, other options, which ironically involve playing more sound. Low-volume white noise, and its softer cousin, pink noise, is an excellent way to block out ambient sounds. It works by playing random sounds at every frequency range except bass and very high treble. Pink noise sounds a lot like the sound of a waterfall. Other sounds are drowned out and there are no easily recognizable sounds such as a voice or instrument for the mind to focus on. We attune to the fuzzy noise and our brains lose focus on any specific sound allowing us to avoid distraction.

If working in a noisy environment is unavoidable for you, we recommend going to YouTube to find either pink noise or the sound of a waterfall and playing it on earphones whilst you work. Adjust the volume to just the right level to cut out any background noise, but not too loud to be distracting.

There are other options to avoid distracting sounds, such as wearing noise-canceling headphones or even by being in an environment such as a library where silence is the rule.

Research into office environments in Hong Kong showed that sound, in particular, causes employees' distraction and annoyance, which results in low productivity. Hundreds of staff complained about the difficulty of focusing attention in their busy offices.[171]

For anyone who attended college, you will know that the library is a sacred place where no sound is allowed – certainly not in the reading space, anyway. This is the space where students retreat to craft their best work because they know just how much more productive it will be. Many students will also know the feeling of working in the middle of the night, and although the reason for this is usually down to too much partying earlier in the term, it's very apparent that the silence is extremely helpful. We would caution, however, that fighting your circadian rhythm is futile. At 2 a.m., your body is asleep, whether your eyes are open or not.

Real interruptions from people are one thing, but many of us know that it's our own mind that interrupts us the most. Whether our mind wanders to hunger, boredom, or an unresolved argument with a partner, we have a tough time focusing. Self-coaching is a great way to help with this, but it's not the only solution. Remember the advanced chess players who focused their attention more effectively than the novices? How did they become so adept at focusing on the essential element of the game? How did they become experts at information accumulation? The answer may come from the military: drills.

Efficiency Hack 2 | Drills

According to Ole Angel, a former Commander in the Norwegian Navy and a successful corporate player in his own right, the military knows a thing or two about managing energy and it does three things very well indeed. One of the most interesting people you will ever meet Ole's career has included everything from negotiating with hostage takers to selling weapons for the US defense industry and finally to a more altruistic role managing operations for a major renewable energy player. Climbing a remote mountain in a new country every year and with an office overlooking a stunning Norwegian fjord, it's safe to say that Ole lives his life to the fullest. We were keen to learn from Ole how the military manages fatigue. Military personnel may be required to go for long extended periods without rest, yet still be able to function at the highest level. Unlike for most of us, the stakes in that game can be life and death.

The first common practice is napping. Short 20 to 30-minute bursts of sleep to be taken whenever the opportunity arises. The second practice is working to what's called, "surplus time." The military knows that when there is a deadline to meet, all manner of things that can happen – will happen, in what's known in the military as the friction of war. For that reason they work to achieve the tasks in the shortest time possible, long before the deadline. They also know, that this will allow them the capacity to take opportunities that may present themselves on the battlefield.

The third practice Ole shared with us is just how heavily the military focuses on drills – drills for how to think and act in a wide range of scenarios, from reloading a rifle to rapidly assessing injured soldiers for priority treatment whilst under enemy fire. Unlike most corporations, the military does not throw good people into a situation and hope for the best. The military practices relentlessly until the skills needed, both mental and physical, become what is known in learning psychology as an "unconscious competence." Unconscious competence is the ability to perform a skill without the need for thinking through the activity step by step. Our expert chess players had unconscious competence at assessing the key elements of the game and ignoring its irrelevant aspects. If you drive a car, you should have the unconscious competence to operate the gears, brakes and steering without having to concentrate on those actions.

Professional athletes share a lot in common with the military. Professional sportsmen and women perform drills and specific plays tirelessly, far and above the level that the average person could possibly hope to achieve, and they do this at competition levels of concentration and perfection.

Take, for example, a weekend warrior golf player who may hit 200 practice balls, hacking away at each one and quickly moving to the next. With each new ball, he thinks about one small aspect of his swing and ignores the rest. Enjoying a beer with his buddies and chatting away with his fellow players, he annihilates 200 practice balls in 30 minutes. Golf practice for the weekend warrior is a social engagement, and that's fine, of course, but there are better ways to improve your game.

This is not how professional players approach practice. Each shot is treated as a competition shot, complete with the mental and physical routine you typically see pro-players work though when you watch them in tournaments on television. The professional player works much harder too, getting through more than 300 practice balls in a morning. The drills mean that, in competition, the player doesn't need to think about each swing; they can focus on the important parts of competition, like staying calm and focused on the critical elements of the game just like our expert chess players. In short – total immersion.

Some competitors take it further and manage to get into the zone. To quote world champion figure skater Owen Edwards in interview with us once again:

> *"I'd say that this one is hard to describe. It's like something beyond consciousness. I think a non-sports person would liken it to intense concentration, but for me it actually isn't. I don't actually think about anything, not the steps, not the routine, not the performance or the technique required, or even how you feel physically... it's more of an awareness of yourself at that point in time. I think it stems from a confidence and belief in your preparation. After all, if you have trained hard your body can perform what you need to do through muscle memory alone. You don't really hear the outside stuff, the fans, etc., it's tuned out. It's just about being calm, relaxed, but knowing you are ready to do your job."*

The key takeaway is the training and drills. Performed over many years, the drills have allowed Owen to move through his competition performances focused only on awareness and without consciously thinking about each move and twist. At that moment, Owen is as efficient as he could possibly be with his energy. Only drills can make that happen.

So what drills can we practice in our jobs and everyday lives that would help us to access a state of deep immersion, feeling more energized and even connected?

Clearly each drill is personal and situation-specific. In our years of leadership training, we have drilled managers in how to assess leadership scenarios and to choose the right leadership style for the situation without having to think too much about it. If we don't drill to a level of unconscious competence, they are likely to go back to their old ways of doing things and the training would be for nothing. Better to drill them in the classroom where they can try, fail, and learn. This allows the manager to automatize otherwise complex and sometimes counter-intuitive skills.

For a sporting or skill-based endeavor, the drills must relate to the precise discipline, i.e., golf, making music, or even administration. Most people will be well drilled in how to use the basic equipment, e.g., the golf clubs or music software, but few people go further than that. The advanced chess players were well drilled in how to make the specific moves of a pawn or queen, for example, but they were also well drilled on how to quickly assess the key elements of the game. Ignoring and inhibiting unnecessary visual scanning of the chessboard, they are accumulating only the strategic information.

For more ubiquitous everyday situations, where we simply want a little more head-space and mental energy left to perform well in anything we do, we may want to drill for and automatize a more general skill, such as problem solving, thinking win/win, active listening, or even empathizing. Here is a list of drills for everyday ubiquitous situations:

- Identifying critical success factors
- Self-coaching
- Win/win thinking
- Empathy
- Active listening
- Staying calm under pressure
- Critical thinking
- Problem solving

To give you an example of an everyday drill we have used to success to the level of automatization, we'll take win/win thinking. It's ideal in that it can be applied in the office, at home, or otherwise in a wide range of situations. It's also a very positive skill which will lead to less conflict and therefore higher levels of vitality. Here's how it's done.

First, we detailed the particular sequence of the skill on paper:

1. What do [they] want?
2. What do I/we want?
3. What's the big picture?
4. What's the solution?

Next, practice your drill at home in a range of imaginary scenarios, maybe imagining your manager, family or friends. Reflect on what's easy and difficult each time and what you can do to improve the method. Build the drill into a daily practice, actively seeking out practice opportunities as they arise throughout your day. You could be at the supermarket checkout and, imagining a win/win with the hard working cashier: What does the cashier want? What do I want? What's the environment and big picture? What's the win/win solution?

It's a simple drill which we tested by performing five times each morning and then in practice throughout the day, for a period of weeks. In order to help with behavior change, and to make the drill stick, follow the exercise regimen and diet hacks in this book *and* lead a self-assessment of how the new skill will benefit you personally. Many of the hacks in this book help to support neuroplasticity which is the brain's ability to be flexible and adaptable to new skills. The self-contemplation step is essential, as we discussed in an earlier chapter. Self-contemplation, as we know, activates the part of the prefrontal cortex (PFC) that's responsible for behavior change. The key is to assess how good or bad an activity is *for you* and not how it is good or bad *in general*. For example, the statement, "Cigarettes are bad," has less behavior-changing effect than, "Cigarettes are bad *for me*."

What drills can you develop? Follow this five-step process to identify and develop a drill tailored just for you:

1. Think about your life right now. What one soft skill do you wish you had, that would take your life to the next level? E.g. assertiveness, empathy etc. Write it down.
2. Break the skill down into simple practicable steps and practice in imaginary scenarios until you are comfortable with the sequence.
3. Practice the skill in real scenarios, with real people as often as you can throughout your day. It can also help to make it into a game, by counting the number of times per day you practiced and beating your personal best.
4. After each practice self reflect, "What did I learn from this practice? and, "In what ways is this skill good for me personally?"
5. Congratulate yourself for taking the time to practice the skill and celebrate any successes. This step will hack the dopamine system to help form a new habit..
6. Repeat daily for at least 30 days.

Training and drills need to be hot, live-fire exercises where the skills are not only practiced, but they are practiced in realistic conditions – or as close to realistic as possible. Most people can easily do the win/win drill in a car or sitting on the sofa, but when we sit down at an important business meeting we're likely to remember to use the skill when we leave the room. Fortunately, this can be hacked. We can create the live-fire practice exercise by re-creating distraction and stress. This will make our information accumulation skills much sharper.

Think about your own drill and see how you can take it up a level. Maybe do it in a busy bar or restaurant; maybe watch a movie with headphones and turn the volume up. Whatever it takes, the results will pay off big time when the moment comes for the real performance. You will more easily be able to enter a state of flow with surplus energy for concentration for the critical aspects of your game. We guarantee that your opponent, whether in sports or in business, or just your 3 year old son, will be at a distinct disadvantage if you are able to focus your precious energy resources on the strategic aspects of your chosen engagement. It will prove a competitive advantage for you.

Efficiency Hack 3 | Work to a Timer

Working to a timer is a good idea, not because of the rest period that follows, which is of course quite useful, but because of its magical effect on focus. As we have seen so far in this book, the notion that the brain needs a rest period may be somewhat more prosaic than we first thought since the brain is always on, functioning at a very high level in either inhibitory or excitatory mode. Technically, what we are really talking about when we reference mental fatigue is *boredom* and losing focus.

Studies have long since demonstrated that we can only pay full attention for 20 minutes at a time at most.[172] Although this is true, when studying, people often attempt to process lots of data over long periods of time. While that might efficiently put the information in front of the learner, it actually decreases the chances the learner will absorb it. The brain will lose focus unless its attention is recaptured roughly every 20 minutes (or less).

What happens in the brain when we lose and then recapture attention? There are actually two separate systems of the brain that interact with one another. One is driven by goals and intentions and is called the dorsal attention network. It serves the function of directing our attention toward something we choose to focus on. The second system, called the ventral attention network, is triggered by stimuli from the external world and takes away any focus.[173] Think of this as a type of "system refresh." While it might be tempting at times to wish that the "system refresh" could be disabled so that we could stay focused for longer, it would actually not be beneficial. The two systems are more like a phone and its charger. One without the other doesn't really get the job done. The reason for this synchronicity is that the things around us naturally change moment- to-moment and we need the capacity both to detect when the world has changed and also to refresh each of the brain's systems so that our attention can refocus optimally. The ventral system grabs our attention when something changes in the environment – especially when unexpected – making it possible for us to react more effectively. Meanwhile, the dorsal system that's responsible for focus, gets a chance to refresh and refocus on other novel stimuli if we so choose.

While the interplay between the dorsal and ventral systems helps explain why attention tends to shift around rather than staying put, a separate mechanism may also be at play. Whenever we put effort into inhibiting our impulses, that effort tends to fatigue various executive functions.[174] Suppose you are trying to stay focused on a lecturer who has been talking for a while. It seems reasonable to suggest you would find yourself frequently inhibiting the urge to glance around the room, to check email on your phone, or to tune out the distracting noise from construction work outside. Perhaps you would find yourself politely attempting to inhibit the desire to move or to interrupt and ask the lecturer to get to the point. You may even find yourself lost in thought about what happened the day before, when suddenly you are called upon in a pop quiz–like fashion and find yourself in need of inhibiting those memories of the day before and directing your cognitive effort to focus on the information you need to recall in order to answer well. These – all forms of inhibition – are likely to rely to some degree on a single prefrontal brain region that has been dubbed "the brain's braking system." [175] [176] [177] Continually putting the brakes on oneself, constantly exercising self-control, is likely to mentally wear you out.

In the brain, the additional focus created by the PFC will, via the rostrum brainstem, suppress the perception of incoming sound and allow you to focus on your work.[178] Similar to mindfulness, working to a timer is great training in concentration and the kind you need to enter the immersive flow state for optimal productive use of your energy.

Breaks are recommended when a sustained level of attention is at stake. Optimally, these breaks won't last more than 10 minutes. It is, of course, very personal, and there will be times for some people, when you can focus optimally for longer periods and need less breaks. This naturally happens when our interest is high or we are under the pressure of a deadline and this is why the artificial deadline of a timer works so well.

When you're in flow you don't want to be interrupted. Flow is where the magic happens; it's that deep immersed concentration where we are completely at one with the task at hand. When work is broken by a timer and you're still deep in the flow state, hitting repeat on the timer for one more round, without taking the break, may be optimal.

Our advice is to use the timer as a tool to train your mind to concentrate in highly distracting environments. This is a powerful energy hack. Together with mindfulness training, this will help you to strengthen the synaptic connections that inhibit external sounds, which allows full concentration on the task. We believe that it is as important to be efficient with our energy as it is to generate more of it. Working to a timer is a great place to start.

Efficiency Hack 4 | Tracking

It is often said that, "What gets measured improves," and there is evidence of this throughout our lives, both in business and science. Many years ago, a high school principal once confided a quite astonishing discovery that he had made whilst managing the payroll of his vast college. Bill, a tall, skinny man with a taste for avant guard jazz, he was an ex teacher himself. One of his favorite phrases , "what gets measured gets improved," was used as defensive jab to anyone who dared to inquire to the reason that the college had a whole department dedicated to generating and processing time sheets for part-time contracted teachers. The process seemed unnecessary, bureaucratic and wasteful. It transpired that several other large colleges had discovered that when they switch to using this time-sheet system, complete with multiple layers of authorizing signatures, their monthly payroll, the amount they were spending each month dropped by a staggering 33%. Fraudulent time-sheet submission was clearly a major issue. With over 15,000 teachers at the college, that amounts to a whole lot of mis-spent money that could otherwise have been spent on high-value facilities, more teaching staff and all of the things that transform the lives of students.

Bill's mantra, "what gets measured, improves," stayed with us ever since. It naturally followed that when we started to think about our own precious energy as a resource, we were curious to discover where we might be spending it too.

We decided to track our energy usage using the simple tracker shown below.

Energy Tracker

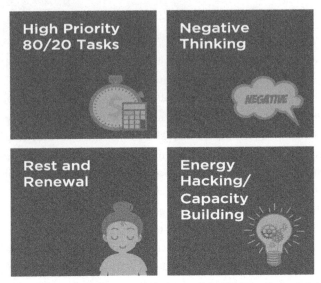

Our tracking system has four quadrants. The first quadrant is labeled "80/20 Tasks." Naturally we were curious as to the amount of our attention and energy was being spent on the things that really move our lives forward, versus the procrastination that most of us default to at some point during our day.

Pareto's Principle, otherwise known as the 80/20 rule, will be well known to many readers. The rule stipulates that 80% of the results come from 20% of the activities. As people of science, we prefer not to go with pop culture and cliches but this one came with some illustrious backing. At a meeting with a highly successful entrepreneur and founder of a global fashion chain, we were given a lesson. The well known fashion designer, reclining in a wicker chair on the terrace of his stunning tropical home was proud to share some of the wisdom that had made him successful: "I've created 2 separate billion dollar companies from scratch. I can tell you, 80/20, that's the key to success."

Of course, we were aware of the 80/20 rule, but we'd never really applied it until then. Our own results, although not yet resulting in a billion dollar company, have been extremely positive to say the least and that's why we were keen to add it as a quadrant to the energy tracker.

We labeled the next quadrant "Negative Thinking," which includes expecting the worse, dissing the boss, and arguing with people in those pointless imagined arguments that you will never actually have. Those pointless imagined arguments are often linked to an external locus of control and a futile search for external validation. Maybe not an entirely optimal use of our precious energy and the brain's resources but they can offer a clue to where we need to take more control and to re-frame our situation more positively as we discussed in a previous section.

The third quadrant is, "Rest and Renewal." As we know, one of the reasons that we feel tired and lethargic after concentrating for long periods is that our neurotransmitter re-uptake has its limits and needs to recuperate. We also know that taking a 20-minute nap, especially at the circadian dip time, is a tried and tested strategy used by the military on long missions; as confided to use by our Norwegian Naval Commander, Ole Angel who we mentioned earlier too. Renewal could include a nap, going for a walk, taking a break, or spending time with the family. The importance here is taking a time to pause and restore.

Capacity building/energy hacking is the fourth quadrant. In this quadrant we refer to time spent exercising, self-coaching, visualizing goals, eating the energy-hacks diet, working to a timer, and adopting all of the other hacks contained in this book.

Putting the tracker to work was life changing. It was revealing how much energy we were wasting on the negative thinking quadrant and how much time we were wasting on procrastinating around the priority 80/20 tasks. You know that something is effective when even your team members approach to ask where you've found so much energy recently. Suffice to say that the energy tracker was a breakthrough for us but before we go into the results and the tactics, it's important to know why the energy tracker works from a neuroscience perspective.

The success of the energy tracker lies once again with the dopamine system and the phenomenon of behavior change through feedback. Since Pavlov studied a few dogs way back in the late 19th century, we have known that behavior can be changed with conditioning. Although that famous experiment was to prove the idea of learned helplessness (i.e., that at some point we simply give up), the notion of operant conditioning comes from the reward we get from performing a specific, hopefully beneficial action.

It's worth reminding ourselves here about our elegant dopamine system. When we perform an action with the promise of a reward, several systems are activated including the dopamine system and the striatal neurons, each serving a different function which add up to modifying our behavior in response to a reward.[179]

The dopamine neurotransmitter, as we have seen, is one of the most important for positive energy and motivation and is largely controlled by the midbrain, with lots of receptors in the PFC. The role of dopamine and the striatal neurons in our evolution cannot be understated, as they are responsible for reward learning, which is a sequential process. It begins with scanning the environment for a possible reward, assessing the potential value of the reward, taking action to attain the object, assessing the reward, and then modifying our neuronal connections accordingly.

The outcome is that prehistoric man was able to constantly update his preferences in response to his changing environment, thus conserving his energy and keeping him alive. The dopamine system is responsible for the scanning of the environment and assessing the value of the reward, i.e., assessing whether it was worth the effort or not, and then modifying our memory; and the striatal system is responsible for taking that information and controlling our behavior. It is another delightfully elegant example of how our brains have evolved and it is one of the key ways that we differ from birds and other non-primates.

It's worth knowing that if we have previously failed to receive the reward, especially if it was promised, the effect is greatly diminished. This phenomenon is called the "reward prediction error." If the reward does not match our expectations, our dopamine system is less activated and we learn not to waste our energy again. If, however, our expectations are exceeded, our dopamine system is significantly activated and we learn to invest our energy in that action again. This learning system is amongst the many functions that dopamine serves that have helped us to evolve into the species we are today.[180] It is also the reason why the energy tracker is so effective.

This is the neural basis for Pavlov's "operant conditioning." Operant conditioning is one of the most basic forms of learning that involves getting some kind of reward for performing a specific action. Think lab rats pushing on a lever to get a food reward. This, however, is only half the story.

Researchers wired the brains of rats undergoing operant conditioning to find out what was really happening as they embarked on their tiny learning curves. The researchers found that two areas of the brain showed synaptic changes. The less active of the two regions was the hippocampus, which we associate with memory;

the surprise was that the area of the brain that showed the biggest increased in synaptic strength was the ventral medial prefrontal cortex (vmPFC).[181]

The answer, therefore, to why our simple tracker is so effective lies in the energy-hungry PFC, specifically the vmPFC. This is the part of the brain sitting just behind the eyes that researchers say is responsible not only for learning but for *behavior change* – the kind that we see in the operant-conditioned lab rats.[182] Indeed, research suggests that activation of this area is a *predictor* of behavior change.

In humans, the dopamine neurons in the vmPFC play a role in *self-related processing* and positive evaluation, specifically with regards to social and cultural factors as well as values (i.e., when we modify our behaviors because of the reactions of others). The irony of the fact is that the brain is actually more interested in its own survival than that of others, so when it evaluates situations based on the social impact, it confirms that our social nature is essential for our survival.

There is evidence of a curious effect that occurs when we assess our actions and behaviors relative to ourselves rather than conceptually. The vmPFC is far more active when we assess whether something is actually good or bad for us as opposed to being conceptually good or bad, which may go a long way in explaining the powerful effects of coaching and why coaching has been described as self-directed neuroplasticity.

As we mentioned earlier, researchers found that when subjects were asked to assess whether smoking, for example, was "good" or "bad" *in general,* far less of the vmPFC was activated than when they were asked whether or not smoking was good for them *personally.* This crucial change in perspective is the key to behavior change. We use self-reflection as a tool for achieving behavior change in all of our training events by simply asking the question, "In what ways is this good for you personally?"

The self-reflection of scoring our energy usage, and the increase in synaptic strength within the vmPFC, is the reason that our simple energy tracker very quickly changed our behavior to the desired result.

Try our energy tracker for one week and see how focused and efficient you are with your energy. Enjoy your new found level of vitality.

The "Negative Thinking" Quadrant

We want to give special attention to the negative thinking quadrant of the energy tracker. We know that many readers are reading this book because you may be currently feeling fatigued and would like to take control of your energy and vitality. We also know that negative thinking is common for many people suffering the effects of fatigue and also the state of emotional burnout. If that's you, you're certainly not alone.

Negative thinking is an energy vampire which seems to take up an extraordinary amount of our time and energy. Negative thinking, or pathological pessimism, as it is sometimes referred to, has its roots in the right hemisphere of the brain, while positive thinking has its roots on the left side.[183] Negative thinking is associated with depression and anxiety, two sides of the same coin and both associated with fatigue and low levels of energy and vitality.

We should caution here that a little negativity can be a good thing if it keeps us in balance. Although we prescribe positive psychology as an energy hack, it should be noted that we don't mean "magical thinking." Magical thinking is where we set a goal so high or unrealistic that we line ourselves up for failure and disappointment should the reward not match our expectations. Positive psychology is about optimism, and optimism is not about framing all situations as winnable; it's about not viewing all defeats as inevitable. It's also about an internal locus of control.

Of course, in the real world, we will always come across problems which cause us anxiety. The power lies in the left brain. Practicing mindfulness to identify your thoughts and emotions and then self-coaching to problem-solve are both left brain activities. This approach prevents negative thinking from becoming destructive and prevents the creative right brain from blowing the problem out of all proportion. An incredibly simple left-brain hack may lie in simply squeezing a ball in the right hand.

Researchers use this technique when they want to stimulate and study the left brain, as the left brain controls the right side of the body. A fascinating byproduct of this phenomenon is that persistence and determination are controlled by our left brain too, and simply squeezing the ball with your right hand may calm your negative thoughts as well as increase your determination by as much as 60%.[184]

One of the effects of negative thinking is that it makes you feel tired and lethargic. Although the reasons are not clear, the effect certainly is. This is, of course, highly dependent on the problem, the individual, whether the individual has a natural problem-solving ability, and their level of self-esteem. Most of us on occasion turn molehills into mountains, and some tend to do the opposite. Self-coaching and thinking through possible solutions to the problem is the key here, as has been shown in the famed experiments of psychologist Martin Seligman, one of the first people to propose the idea of positive psychology.

Seligman studied learned helplessness, which is the state in which a person feels that they are powerless to evade an unpleasant situation even when a solution exists. It can be likened to a pessimistic viewpoint that things will never change. Although Seligman's early experiments were on dogs, his later experiments on humans proved to be compelling. In one such experiment, participants were given a test to perform while a loud distracting noise wailed in their ears.[185] One group had access to a lever which would stop the noise if pulled; the other did not. The surprise finding was that the group that had the lever understandably fared better in their tests, but in a twist of logic, they did not all pull the lever. It seemed that merely knowing that the option was there was enough to improve mental focus on the task.

Negative thinking, therefore, can be overcome with simple self-coaching to the point that multiple options are tabled in order to resolve the issue, regardless of whether they are actually followed through with. Tracking the time that you spend on negative thinking will help you to focus on solutions and options rather than the endless rumination and aggravating thoughts that frequently accompany negative thinking.

In essence, it takes back the locus of control which, according to research, may be hardwired into us. As we mentioned, research indicates that those with a more optimistic outlook have higher left hemisphere activation and those with a pessimistic outlook had greater right hemisphere activation. The locus of control, as we know, is what psychologists call our predisposition to judge events around us as either within our control or out of our control. In essence, self-coaching, and coaching in general, helps to take back that locus of control. An internal locus of control is the ideal state for higher energy and vitality, because with it we can act with commitment and confidence that our energy will not go to waste. For a more detailed explanation of how to self-coach, you can revisit the section on of self-coaching in the neuro-hacks chapter of this book.

So, in conclusion, using our energy tracker (or even one of your own) can help to increase your energy levels and vitality by employing the dopamine system, the vmPFC, and striatal neurons, in modifying the behaviors that will help you to win and to achieve the results that you want. The feeling of achieving your goals is vitalizing, and the tracker will help you to stay focused on developing your energy and using it well. Increasing your self-discipline, and nurturing the internal locus of control will help you to feel more energy in your life. Happy tracking!

Efficiency Hack 5 | Task Switching: Putting the Hardest First

Interruptions sap our energy. Diversion of our attentional resources is sometimes referred to by psychologists as 'task switching,' especially in relation to work tasks. As you can imagine, much research has gone into task switching over the years. Task switching utilizes more mental resources, results in more mistakes, and takes longer, which ultimately leads to frustration. Indeed, in one study, after only 20 minutes of interrupted performance, people reported significantly higher stress, frustration, workload, effort, and pressure.[186]

One model of attention and processing in the brain suggests that when we perform a task that we are familiar with (brushing your teeth with your right hand) and then switching to a task we are unfamiliar with (brushing your teeth with your left hand), the brain must first actively suppress the first skill and actively concentrate on applying a new skill. This is another kind of task switching, and the evidence suggests that going from something we know well to something we are less unfamiliar with takes more time and therefore more energy. Although this sounds obvious, it suggests a possible energy hack. If the brain uses more energy to switch from a familiar task to a less familiar task, you can start your day with the hardest and most unfamiliar tasks before moving on to the more repetitive and familiar tasks. For example, if tax reporting (or authoring a book) isn't your regular thing, do this task before moving on to the tasks you do more regularly. Cascade accordingly.

Efficiency Hack 6 | Pause and Restore

No matter what the profession or skill, most people would agree that before a big presentation, a big test, a big race or any other challenge, the best way to prepare yourself is to be in a good place mentally, to be well rested, properly fed, and fully committed. But, in what ways is this relevant to the regular challenges we face daily? Whilst we know our muscles need to be rested, we also know the neurons in our brain need to recharge too, yet we are often reluctant to give our *mind* the same opportunity? By mind we refer to consciousness, sensing, thinking and perceiving. The mind is easily the most incredible part of our body, whilst at the same time, it continues to be the least understood in science.

If you aim to gain muscle mass you exercise, eat protein and lift weights. What is fascinating is that your muscles actually do not grow during exercise but actually after you work-out. Your body repairs damaged muscle fibers that were used during the work-out by fusing them together to form new muscle protein strands or myofibrils[187]. These repaired myofibrils increase in thickness and number to create muscle growth.

Likewise, when you aim to learn new information, this process doesn't actually happen while you study and read. It is not until you sleep that the information you learned is properly coded into your long term memory[188]. This time-lapse between actions and results is not considered a resting period, they are not moments of inactivity but active moments of change. Similarly, our mind needs moments of pausing its normal activity and restoring. Not to be confused with idly doing nothing, but on the contrary, purposefully seeking balance.

Restoring our state of mind is essential to achieving our fullest energy potential. It is about that deep breath before the fight, that inner peace that keeps our cool, having a moment for yourself, to rethink, relax, renew, redirect and recollect. This mind restoration can be achieved in many ways, not in vain it has been at the heart of an endless list of fads and practices throughout history. From the relaxation complexes in the Palace at Knossos dated mid-second millennium BC, to current relaxation apps, humans are constantly seeking ways to achieve optimal mental rest.

Restoring is a step ahead from resting. It is not about recharging an energy level like a smartphone's battery, but reinstating balance. Whether it is yoga, meditation, journal writing, a short walk, praying, reading a good book or feeling a song; having a period of time every day where you are focused on some level of introspection is highly beneficial. Finding a space for relaxed breathing and peace is essential for restoration. Many activities aim at reaching self-regulation or a heightened level of consciousness. Nonetheless, not every activity is for anyone. What might be fulfilling for many might be draining for others. It is important you take the time to discover what is restoring for you personally. For example, many extroverts enjoy resting periods the most when they do them with other people.[189]

Two of the most common restoring activities nowadays include yoga and mindfulness. There is a tendency to pack yoga, meditation and mindfulness into one concept. The truth is that meditation is not really a synonym of silence, control breathing, and mindfulness. Technically speaking, mindfulness is a subcategory of meditation pinpointing on the idea of being completely focused on the present moment. Yoga is actually a physical, mental and spiritual discipline dating back to the fifth century BC that at its origins seeks to unify the human spirit and the divine in Hinduism tradition. In pop culture, yoga has been almost fully stripped from its spiritual origins and blended into gymnastics, resulting in a modern adaptation that strikes more as a discipline rooted in the achievement of physical postures and breath control. In pop culture or in religious practice, research suggests yoga might produce many medical benefits. Beyond its spiritual origins, yoga has demonstrated to have beneficial health effects. Looking at over 3517 trial participants, doctors have found practicing yoga with breathing techniques and meditation/mental relaxation 3 times a week has a significant impact on blood pressure health[190]. It has also been suggested that yoga has other medical benefits including stress relief[191], anxiety management[192], and chronic disease symptom management[193,194]. The benefits of yoga occur when the physical exercise includes meditation and controlled breathing. It has been found that practicing yoga with mindfulness and proper breathing has added benefits beyond just the physical stretching aspects of yoga[195].

Although mindful mediation has thousands of years of history in the Buddhist religion, it's only in the last decade that it has been studied empirically. The popularity of secular mindfulness programs are partly attributed to the decline of other traditional religions, and as a collateral to the impact of technologies in our personal lives. The practice of mindful meditation can lead to increased happiness, better health, feeling more self-directed and cooperative. This is because mindfulness can help you to think of your life as a narrative in which you play a role, a story in which your actions contribute in a meaningful way to others and yourself.

One of the appeals of mindfulness is that it can be practiced pretty much anywhere, at any time and without the need for equipment. Mindfulness is a natural ability all humans have to be fully aware and present in any particular moment without becoming overwhelmed with circumstances or other factors. Although it is a basic human ability, as with any skill, it can be developed and perfected. Evidence supports that mindfulness reduces stress, enhances performance, helps us to gain insight and awareness through observing what is going on in our own minds and increases our attention to that which surrounds us, both circumstances and sensation[196]. Hence mindfulness has found its way into mainstream science, not only becoming the subject of rigorous scientific research, but also as a therapeutic application to a variety of psychological and medical conditions.

Awareness/focus and acceptance/compassion are the two main types of mindfulness. They both involve focused concentration on our moment-to-moment reality, but acceptance and compassion-based mindfulness also involve modifying our interpretations of sensations and emotions towards a different state, specifically, acceptance, kindness, compassion and being non-judgmental. Research has shown that complimenting meditation practice with a positive emotional component (e.g. acceptance/compassion meditation) cultivates these qualities and increases them accordingly.[197]

The key to mindful mediation is staying present in the moment. Being aware of fast forwarding to the future or rewinding to the past, the goal is simply to stay present in the moment whether you are doing a body-scan or doing the washing up. This level of meditation is the starting point for most people new to meditation and will continue to be the foundation as you move on to other types of meditation which have different functions. Crucially for this section on cognitive efficiency, focus based meditation practice builds the "muscles" that will allow you to stay focused deeper and for longer, allowing you to use your precious energy and vitality with great efficiency on your work, projects or whatever you should choose.

Our recommended mindful mediation for this type of one pointed focus is the body-scan meditation.

The important part of the body-scan meditation is not to try to control any part of your body or to "feel a certain way." The mindset is simply to accept any sensations with focused curiosity e.g. if your foot feels cold, so be it, just notice how cold it is. The purpose is to develop a level of concentration that will allow you to ignore, and not interact with, negative unhelpful thinking and to learn to just accept things as they are without needing to control everything.

Before we take you through the steps of the body-scan meditation, a skill that can help you to reach a mindful state is learning to label your thoughts. Labeling your thoughts is also a powerful life skill for emotional stress which involves observing your thoughts as they enter your consciousness and then simply labeling them as "stress," "worry," "anxiety," "happiness," etc., but not following the train of thought further. This may surprise you greatly, but you really don't have to interact with every thought that enters your mind in the same way that you don't open every email in your inbox, some of it is just spam!

You can use thought labeling as part of your body scan meditation. Here's how it works:

1. Lie down somewhere quiet where you will not be disturbed.

2. Close your eyes and focus on breathing in through your nose, note the feeling of air as it touches your nostrils, note the temperature, the sounds and all other sensations.

3. Random thoughts will enter your mind, and they will include your emotions and thoughts about the stressors in your life. Without actually engaging with, or following, a train of thoughts, simply label each thought e.g. That's thinking, that's anxiety, that's

stress. Once labeled, focus all of your attention back on breathing through your nose.

4. Next, move the focus of your attention down your body to your big toe. Take a note of the sensation of the toe touching your sock or the feeling of air as it touches the skin. Move attention to the next toe and notice the sensations in the same way. Move to the next toe. Pay as much attention as you can to each toe and then move to the sole of the foot, noting the sensations. If you can feel the pulsation of the heart beating through your toes you've nailed it, but this could take a few sessions.

5. Move your focus to the entire foot and hold the whole foot in awareness, paying attention to all of the sensations you feel there.

6. Move on to the leg and repeat the same process of focusing on smaller areas of the leg in great detail and with curiosity and finally holding the whole leg in awareness. Repeat this process throughout the body for the other foot, leg, the back, the groin and genital area, the tummy and stomach area, the chest, the shoulders, the arms and hands and the head. Finally, hold the whole body in awareness. The whole bodyscan should take around 30 minutes.

Self-awareness of the thoughts that enter your mind and your true emotional state is the foundation of the longer-term solutions to emotional stress management, specifically the triggers. Once you have the ability to see patterns of thoughts and emotions, you can begin to write them down and try to understand your thought patterns in an objective way. In a mindfulness context, the key to accepting our strong emotions is to create what's called a "safe container." This has many forms. Firstly, it's a specific time and appropriate place to accept your strong emotions such as anger or disappointment. The best safe container is to have a supportive group of friends and family who you can share your deepest emotions with in a healthy way. Your ability to master the focus/

awareness mediations is the first step. Without the ability to become aware of your emotions you will not have the sensitivity to pick up on the signals which represent your suppressed emotions.

Although mindfulness and compassion are complementary practices, and can work in mutually reinforcing ways[198] , it must be said that breath-focused meditation practices or activities alone will not necessarily bring changes in compassion, cooperation or other ethical behaviors. Needless to say, explicitly cultivating compassion and other ethical behaviors without meditation will in itself boost these positive outcomes[199][200]. After all, what we practice and fill our days with has a direct impact on our emotional and intellectual pool. What we are exposed to has a direct impact as to how we perceive the world. Practicing compassion in mindful meditation provides an excellent practice area to learn to experience the emotion of compassion and to strengthen those pathways. As with any skill practice, the real world "on the job" application in our day to day lives further strengthens the skill until it becomes automatic and native to us.

Priming is an excellent way we have evolved to become more receptive to positive emotions, including compassion. The effects of priming are well studied in the scientific community. Your brain is wired to take cues from context and associate them with what it knows. The most simple associative and context priming effects can be seen by rapidly processing target words[201] when reading a sentence[202] or a list of words. For example, if we want you to think about dogs without mentioning the word we can say: puppy, pet, wag, collar, canine, walks, playful. The context is predisposing you to the thought of the word dog, to an extent that you might even recollect hearing the word dog with a high level of certainty, although it was never named[203]. This also applies to the likes of kindness. When a subject experiences an act of kindness, they subsequently experience a lower threshold of activation when encountering a positive stimuli. After being on the receiving end of an act of kindness, you experience a temporarily increased resistance to negative stimuli in addition to the increase activation of positive associative networks.[204]

This is also true for restoring. We can visualize our brain waking up after a good night sleep as a clean slate ready to conquer the world. As the day goes by it gets dirtier and dirtier and dirtier still. In this lineal fashion, we would hit rock bottom by the end of the day, feeling impatient, fatigued and irritable. Taking time to clear our mind and restoring our clean slate is best practice towards assuring healthy inner peace and a feeling of vitality. Restoring is a way to achieve proper emotion regulation, focus and well-being. By directing our attention to the present, especially toward present positive experiences (e.g. restoring activities), there is an increase in intensity and frequency of positive emotions. [205]

Last but not least, engaging in vividly remembering or anticipating positive events has shown to predict well-being and reduce anxiety. [206] [207]

Yoga meditation has gained global popularity amongst a wide group of practitioners only in the last century, Yoga as a religious practice however, has been around for centuries as a source of restoration and this is true for most religions. Historically, in each of the major religions, there are specific practices used to find inner peace and restoration which date back centuries.

For readers who follow a religion, research has shown that endorsing a religion or spirituality can have a positive impact on well-being[208]. As we know from studies in positive psychology, specific positive emotions including awe, gratitude, love and peace are linked to feelings of wellbeing and these emotions are often promoted in many religious practices.

The purpose here is certainly not to promote religion as an energy hack, merely to illustrate that there are practices that have been developed over centuries that tap into our innate need to find inner balance, indicating that inner balance is a fundamental human need. It is also fascinating to observe how practices have developed historically to fulfill those needs that we now know to have a strong correlation human health and wellbeing. Yoga, in particular, is a fascinating example of this but there are others too.

Self transcendence is another great example. Most religions have a transcendent component and share the search for a higher meaning of self. Whilst all positive emotions are beneficial to us, we now know that some allow for greater benefits in terms of well-being. Self-transcendent promotes perspective taking and pro-social behaviors, that we know to be particularly apt at promoting well-being through what's called 'feedback loops.'[209]

Another element that many religions have in common is the recitation and repetition of sounds, words or sentences to aid concentration. Whether it is reciting the Ave Maria or a mantra, these elements enhance and synchronize cardiovascular rhythms[210]. Most of these recitations slow respiration to almost six respirations per minute, which is essentially the same timing as our internal circulatory rhythm. This explains why the practice of controlled breathing, meditation, relaxation and potentially even prayer have long term benefits to blood pressure. Although at first it might seem like this might be a coincidence, there is evidence that links the recitation of mantras and the current structure of the rosary from the Catholic faith. The rosary is a sequence of prayers which is also represented as beads on a necklace. There is historical evidence that the rosary was introduced to Europe by the crusaders, who took it from the Arabs, who learned it from Tibetan monks and the yoga masters of India. This timeline and geographical journey serve as proof that the breathing patterns of these recitations share a common ancestry that spans religious and spiritual practices, geographies and centuries. Maybe the most fascinating things for us however, is the fact that these highly beneficial breathing patterns reflect precisely what we now know in science to be the precise pace of rhythmic breathing to induce calming relaxation response in the body.

The benefits of respiratory exercises to slow respiration in the practice of controlled breathing and recitation of 6 breaths/min, have long been reported. This leads many to believe that many religious practices where cultivated as a device to slow respiration, improve concentration, and induce calm. Breathing at around 10 seconds per breath for 20 minutes a day reduces self-reported stress and anxiety.[211]

Breathing also influences our brain rhythms. The brain regions associated with emotion regulation are one of the areas that have a higher demand for blood flow. Blood flow rhythms are especially likely to impact these areas. Breathing through the nose causes respiration-synced oscillations between the olfactory cortex as well as the amygdala and hippocampus[212]. To recall, the olfactory cortex is the part of the brain responsible for sensations from the nose, and the amygdala can trigger our fight, flight and freeze response. This synchronization therefore controls activity in the brain regions associated with emotion regulation.[213] We know that brain activity is fueled by oxygen transported by blood, so it is only natural that syncing the demands of the emotion regulation centers in the brain with proper blood flow will have a big impact on how well we can regulate our emotions.

Whilst deliberate mindful meditations including yoga are amongst the newest trends and revivals in restoring our balance, there are many other alternative practices that show the same level of benefits. The practice of setting a quiet time that modulates breathing to 6 breaths per minute, improves cognitive performance and enhances emotional regulation[214]. Dedicating time to a meditative state increases activity in the prefrontal cortex and stimulates the reticular nucleus of the thalamus which promotes the secretion of GABA inhibitory molecules, also known as anti-anxiety molecules.[215]

But silence is not the only path towards restoration. Breathing is also highly synced to music. Sounds can induce autonomic responses in listeners. Music not only improves quality of life but also impacts long term changes in heart rate and heart rate variability. Cerebral blood flow has been found to be significantly lower when listening to low tempo classical music compared to high tempo opera. Likewise, music significantly decreases patient's anxiety level in preoperative settings and has proven to work better for this purpose than sedation drugs such as midazolam[216]. Moreover, listening to music while resting in bed after open-heart surgery leads to significant differences in cortisol levels[217]. Not only is it intuitive, but science has proven that there is a strong relationship between subjective and physiological responses to music with a potential to rehabilitate mood, and enhance both wellbeing and quality of life. Although music is most effective for short-term mood enhancement, self-selected music is very effective for inducing a joyous state and restoration.

Our mental state is the frame through which we all live our lives, but it is very easy to get caught in the in the trials and tribulations of life itself. By finding a time and method to pause and restore we allow ourselves to place the clock back at zero, to find perspective, to find new energy with which to achieve our conquests and make sure we do so in the most optimal way possible. Maybe you remember that feeling as a child when you held a freshly sharpened pencil in your hands. You could see how your handwriting and willingness to work was improved just by the fact that there was a refreshed and pristine instrument to work with. Nothing really changed, it was the same tool, but by restoring its sharpness, by optimizing its function, it was a game changer. Make the time to restore your mind, make sure you have a couple of minutes a day to give you the push to be at your best, to find your balance and inner peace, and to nourish your general well-being.

Summary

Being efficient with our energy is as important as generating more of it. The deep and effortless concentration of the immersive 'flow state' is where the magic really happens. It's important to remember also that as humans we respond to the environment that surrounds us in each moment and this in turn determines where our energy if focused. For this reason we need to sharpen the skills to manage our environment, our reaction to it and to frequently restore the imbalances that occur naturally throughout our day with the target being the middle zone of the energy curve.

We learned in this chapter to track our energy using the energy tracker, paying attention to the time spent on negative thinking and the time invested on the stuff that really matters.

We learned in this chapter that sound is one of the biggest distractions at both a conscious and subconscious level and that pink noise, earplugs or a silent place to work go a long way to controlling this distraction. Working to a timer is an excellent way to focus our attention too.

We discovered that the efficient accumulation of information related to the *essence* of a situation is a key skill for energy efficiency and immersion mastery. The ability to effortlessly hone in on the game-winning aspects of any situation, like a grandmaster chess player, frees up cognitive resources and time for assessing choices and making the right decision. The more instinctive we can make the accumulation of key information, the higher our chances of experiencing and enjoying immersive vitality.

The accumulation of the "essence" is a skill that can be drilled in. As we have seen, we can develop drills for any skill and, with the addition of live practice, we can achieve a level of mastery that can take us to new levels in our lives.

By applying the steps in sequence: mastering your environment, focusing your attention and efficiently capturing the essence of situations, we can achieve a level of deep immersion – a free-flowing state of natural energy and vitality.

Remember to do the most challenging and unfamiliar tasks first. Doing our most difficult tasks first thing in the day creates an energy-efficient cascade, helping you to fully utilize your energy resources for maximum productivity. Our lives may be busy yet an imagined need to work at an insane pace has, in recent years, become mis-perceived an essential step for life and business success. Productivity trumps effort every time, and you are more productive when you are fresh.

Ultimately, the experience of vitality is an emotional state of well being. Remember to simply take time to pause and refresh. Take the time to slow your breathing to 6 breaths per minute as often as you can throughout your day, breathing through your nose, following both the wisdom of the ancients and of science to enjoy inner peace and vitality.

We hope that you will use some, or all, of these hacks as tools to help you focus your new-found energy to reach the very highest levels of vitality, productivity and achievement in your life. Productivity and time are the keys to making progress and, as we know, the feeling of personal progress is the key to vitality and the energizing happiness we desire.

CONCLUSION

Energy is Life

Life needs energy to exist. Our ability to transform energy into the movement and consciousness that we enjoy is the very definition of what it is to be alive.

Plants, bacteria, animals, and humans all share the ability to break chemical bonds and molecules, transforming them into usable energy. As a general rule, the more complex the organism, the more complex its energy sources and uses are. An animal's ability to transform energy is superior to that of plants, due to its evolutionary need to transform this energy into more complex skills and behaviors than plants can exhibit. What makes human energy more complex than that of any other species is our ability to use it purposefully – i.e., for means beyond survival. We use energy to think, to create, to socialize, to generate value, to convey emotions, to help others, and to give meaning. Our energy destinations are far beyond those of any other species. We use energy not only to exist, but also to manage to get up in the morning for a fruitful day of work and social change. Humans have a need to allocate their energy to thoughts, emotions, and behaviors that transcend ourselves and give value to our lives. Family, friends, work, hobbies, and so on – they all require time and energy. These social and professional aspects of life require mostly brain power, as opposed to basic biological energy. That is why we can have a large mental load on us, feel emotionally drained, and at the same time have the required biological energy levels to run three miles.

All is Connected

With time, science has come to show that all of these factors are intertwined. We know that physical exercise is capable of inducing structural and functional changes in the brain, resulting in biological and psychological benefits. For a couple of decades it has been known that neuroplasticity is our brain's ability to modify itself in response to experience. This ability is found in both children and adults and can involve the strengthening of a synapses, modifying the amount of gray matter as the actual location transfer of a cognitive faculty. A growing body of scientific literature seem to indicate physical exercise might be a neuroplasticity enhancer.

Although the power of exercise to support cognitive function has been demonstrated, it is most interesting to know that these effects could last for considerably more time that we might think. An emerging line of scientific evidence indicates that the effects of exercise are longer lasting than previously thought up, even to the point of affecting future generations. In the past years there has been a rising interest in the field of epigenetics. Epigenetic modifications make reference to heritable changes in gene function that cannot be explained by alterations in the DNA sequence. Current research on epigenetics suggest they are highly influenced by environmental factors like nutrients and physical exercise. If this is so, physical activity and exercise can modulate gene expression through epigenetic alternations.

The connection between all energy quadrants it so outstanding that it has been found that even microbiome could play a role in improving mood and mental health. This is the foundation of the emerging field of *psychobiotics*. It believed beneficial bacteria in our gut can boost mood, reduce brain fog and improve our ability to handle stress and reduce anxiety and depression. Most research in this area are in the early stages but have so far resulted in significant results in animal studies. We will hear much more about these exciting developments in the years to come.

What Now?

The effects of your energy and vitality habits may outlast even you. It is interesting to know that your vitality levels might not just affect how your biology, your psychology, your wellbeing and how you function today. It might affect more than the ability to achieve a life-time goal or to follow through on a healthy diet. It might be more than being able to think positively or reducing your mental load. It may even go as far as affecting your future descendants.

Life is a work of art. The human ability to break down the chemical bonds in food and then use that energy to paint on the canvas of life is extraordinary. There are literally no limits as to how we can choose to use our energy: from traveling to far off lands, to pondering the hidden meaning held within the ever-changing fabric of our lives. It's not to be forgotten that, even though limitless in applications, energy is a finite and precious resource that we cannot afford to waste. In this book, we have shown you how to increase and efficiently utilize this precious resource. Let's put things in perspective. Upgrading the breaks on a car won't transform it into a Ferrari, but keeping the car beautifully maintained will make it feel like new. The car will stay responsive, powerful, enjoyable to drive and it will take you on long and rewarding journeys.

Following the hacks in this book is a lifestyle, not a quick fix. The lifestyle is the accumulation of many vitalizing new habits which, over time, become transformational. More than the sum of its parts, each of the hacks contained in this book can be considered a new habit. Our suggestion to you is that you take positive action to implement all of the hacks in this book in unison. Combining the hacks from the bio quadrant with efficiency and motivational hacks is a quick and powerful method to make significant progress in your life and projects as we have found through coaching and research. Nearly all of the hacks in this book require little active attention and can be considered a passive energizing habit. Eating the right food and drinking more water and actively maintaining your attention on the energy curve and energy tracker (detailed in the neuro hacks and efficiency quadrants) you can expect to enjoy a deeply pleasing vitalization and improved productivity.

Living life is a commitment. With focus and purpose, we can craft the lives that we truly want for ourselves. If we don't consciously make that choice, it will not happen by itself. We the writers have made that commitment. Having a vitality lifestyle is the foundation that allows you to live the life you really want. In this book we have covered the four areas that affect vitality and energy levels. As you can guess by now, it takes more than just addressing the hacks of one area to achieve a proper energy balance, it requires attention in each quadrant. The energy curve is real and procuring a healthy lifestyle is as important as proactively seeking to unburden our mental load through mindfulness and proper motivational energy.

This book has provided you with the most relevant hacks to really enhance your energy levels and to thrive. Nonetheless, you must remember that whilst energy can be hacked and replenished, time cannot. Time is our most precious resource. Choosing to live a vitality lifestyle will not only give you the energy to achieve your dreams, but it will also allow you to live your dreams for longer. With longevity, we have more time to do more with our lives.

It's time to make your choice.

ACKNOWLEDGMENTS

We would like to give our most sincere thanks to all of the athletes, scientists and contributors to this book who have inspired and informed us. We would like to acknowledge the hard work of research scientists in Universities and laboratories around the world whose tireless dedication brings life changing insights into the worlds of neuroscience, psychology and healthcare.

We would like to give a special mention to Melvin William for his help with research at the early stage of the book, Maria Ulfah for graphics and our families and partners for their enduring and loving support.

ABOUT THE AUTHORS

Maite Balda is a Doctor in Neuroscience, licensed psychologist, owner of her own company and a successful journalist. She is an expert in translating academic neuroscience work into articles available for broader audiences.

Maite lives in New York where she balances work and her family of 6 beautiful children.

www.neubuco.com

Russell Potter is a performance coach and leadership trainer, Russell has worked with global brands around the world teaching motivation strategies to leaders and facilitating breakthroughs. Originally from London England, he now resides in Tokyo.

www.motivo-academy.com

REFERENCES

1   Aronoff, S. L., Berkowitz, K., Shreiner, B., & Want, L. (2004). Glucose metabolism and regulation: beyond insulin and glucagon. *Diabetes Spectrum,17*(3), 183-190.

2   Stickel, F., Baumüller, H. M., Seitz, K., Vasilakis, D., Seitz, G., Seitz, H. K., & Schuppan, D. (2003). Hepatitis induced by Kava (Piper methysticum rhizoma). *Journal of hepatology, 39*(1), 62-67.

3   Stanhope, K. L., Schwarz, J. M., Keim, N. L., Griffen, S. C., Bremer, A. A., Graham, J. L., ... & McGahan, J. P. (2009). Consuming fructose-sweetened, not glucose-sweetened, beverages increases visceral adiposity and lipids and decreases insulin sensitivity in overweight/obese humans. The Journal of clinical investigation, 119(5), 1322.

4   O'shea, R. S., Dasarathy, S., & McCullough, A. J. (2010). Alcoholic liver disease. *Hepatology, 51*(1), 307-328.

5   Apte, M. V., Wilson, J. S., & Korsten, M. A. (1997). Alcohol-related pancreatic damage. *Alcohol Health & Research World, 21*(1), 13-20.

6   National, C. G. C. U. (2010). Alcohol Use Disorders: Diagnosis and Clinical Management of Alcohol-Related Physical Complications.

7   Yu, C., Cao, Q., Chen, P., Yang, S., Deng, M., Wang, Y., & Li, L. (2016). An updated dose–response meta-analysis of coffee consumption and liver cancer risk. Scientific reports, 6.

8   Gapstur, S. M., Anderson, R. L., Campbell, P. T., Jacobs, E. J., Hartman, T. J., Hildebrand, J. S., ... & McCullough, M. L. (2017). Associations of Coffee Drinking and Cancer Mortality in the Cancer Prevention Study-II. Cancer Epidemiology and Prevention Biomarkers, cebp-0353.

9   Veltri, K. L., Espiritu, M., & Singh, G. (1990). Distinct genomic copy number in mitochondria of different mammalian organs. Journal of cellular physiology, 143(1), 160-164.

10   Bryant, D. E., Marriott, K. E., Macgregor, S. A., Kilner, C., Pasek, M. A., & Kee, T. P. (2010). On the prebiotic potential of reduced oxidation state phosphorus: the H-phosphinate–pyruvate system. Chemical Communications, 46(21), 3726-3728.

11   Rubin, L.L., and J.M. Staddon. 1999. The cell biology of the blood-brain barrier. *Annu. Rev. Neurosci.* 22:11–28

12   Hurtado-Alvarado, G., Velázquez-Moctezuma, J., & Gómez-González, B. (2017). Chronic Sleep Restriction Disrupts Interendothelial Junctions In The Hippocampus And Increases Blood–Brain Barrier Permeability. Journal Of Microscopy.

13   Wagner, B. A., Venkataraman, S., & Buettner, G. R. (2011). The rate of oxygen utilization by cells. *Free Radical Biology and Medicine, 51*(3), 700-712.

14   Thomson, A. J., Webb, D. J., Maxwell, S. R., & Grant, I. S. (2002). Oxygen therapy in acute medical care: the potential dangers of hyperoxia need to be recognised. *BMJ: British Medical Journal,324*(7351), 1406.

15   Schölvinck, M. L., Howarth, C., & Attwell, D. (2008). The cortical energy needed for conscious perception. Neuroimage, 40(4), 1460-1468.

16 Larson, G. E., Haier, R. J., LaCasse, L., & Hazen, K. (1995). Evaluation of a "mental effort" hypothesis for correlations between cortical metabolism and intelligence. Intelligence, 21(3), 267-278.

17 Parks, R. W., Loewenstein, D. A., Dodrill, K. L., Barker, W. W., Yoshii, F., Chang, J. Y., ... & Duara, R. (1988). Cerebral metabolic effects of a verbal fluency test: a PET scan study. Journal of Clinical and Experimental Neuropsychology, 10(5), 565-575.

18 Steiner, J. L., Murphy, E. A., McClellan, J. L., Carmichael, M. D., & Davis, J. M. (2011). Exercise training increases mitochondrial biogenesis in the brain. Journal of applied physiology, 111(4), 1066-107.

19 Wenz, T. (2013). Regulation of mitochondrial biogenesis and PGC-1α under cellular stress. *Mitochondrion*, 13(2), 134-142.

20 Tsai, H. H., Chang, S. C., Chou, C. H., Weng, T. P., Hsu, C. C., & Wang, J. S. (2016). Exercise Training Alleviates Hypoxia-induced Mitochondrial Dysfunction in the Lymphocytes of Sedentary Males. *Scientific reports*, 6, 35170.

21 Jornayvaz, F. R., & Shulman, G. I. (2010). Regulation of mitochondrial biogenesis. *Essays in biochemistry*, 47, 69-84.

22 Häussinger, D. (1996). The role of cellular hydration in the regulation of cell function. *Biochemical Journal*, 313(Pt 3), 697.

23 Jéquier, E., & Constant, F. (2010). Water as an essential nutrient: the physiological basis of hydration. *European journal of clinical nutrition*, 64(2), 115.

24 Grandjean, A. C., & Campbell, S. M. (2004). Hydration: fluids for life.

25 Ritz, P., & Berrut, G. (2005). The Importance of Good Hydration for Day to Day Health. *Nutrition reviews*, 63(s1).

26 Cian, C., Barraud, P. A., Melin, B., & Raphel, C. (2001). Effects of fluid ingestion on cognitive function after heat stress or exercise-induced dehydration. *International Journal of Psychophysiology*, 42(3), 243-251.

27 Cian, C., Koulmann, N., Barraud, P. A., Raphel, C., Jimenez, C., & Melin, B. (2000). Influences of variations in body hydration on cognitive function: Effect of hyperhydration, heat stress, and exercise-induced dehydration. *Journal of Psychophysiology*, 14(1), 29.

28 Ganio, M. S., Armstrong, L. E., Casa, D. J., McDermott, B. P., Lee, E. C., Yamamoto, L. M., ... & Chevillotte, E. (2011). Mild dehydration impairs cognitive performance and mood of men. *British Journal of Nutrition*, 106(10), 1535-1543.

29 Armstrong, L. E., Ganio, M. S., Casa, D. J., Lee, E. C., McDermott, B. P., Klau, J. F., ... & Lieberman, H. R. (2012). Mild dehydration affects mood in healthy young women. *The Journal of nutrition*, 142(2), 382-388.

30 Patel, A. V., Mihalik, J. P., Notebaert, A. J., Guskiewicz, K. M., & Prentice, W. E. (2007). Neuropsychological performance, postural stability, and symptoms after dehydration. *Journal of athletic training*, 42(1), 66.

31 Jéquier, E., & Constant, F. (2010). Water as an essential nutrient: the physiological basis of hydration. *European journal of clinical nutrition*, 64(2), 115.

32 Raichle, M. E., & Gusnard, D. A. (2002). Appraising the brain's energy budget. *Proceedings of the National Academy of Sciences*, 99(16), 10237-10239.

33 Kuszewski, J. C., Wong, R. H., & Howe, P. R. (2017). Effects of Long-Chain Omega-3 Polyunsaturated Fatty Acids on Endothelial Vasodilator Function and Cognition—Are They Interrelated? *Nutrients*, 9(5), 487.

34 Stough, C., Downey, L., Silber, B., Lloyd, J., Kure, C., Wesnes, K., & Camfield, D. (2012). The effects of 90-day supplementation with the omega-3 essential fatty acid docosa-

hexaenoic acid (DHA) on cognitive function and visual acuity in a healthy aging population. *Neurobiology of aging, 33*(4), 824-e1.

35   Bauer, I., Hughes, M., Rowsell, R., Cockerell, R., Pipingas, A., Crewther, S., & Crewther, D. (2014). Omega-3 supplementation improves cognition and modifies brain activation in young adults. *Human Psychopharmacology: Clinical and Experimental, 29*(2), 133-144.

36   Bangen, K. J., Clark, A. L., Edmonds, E. C., Evangelista, N. D., Werhane, M. L., Thomas, K. R., ... & Delano-Wood, L. (2017). Cerebral Blood Flow and Amyloid-β Interact to Affect Memory Performance in Cognitively Normal Older Adults. *Frontiers in Aging Neuroscience, 9*, 181.

37   Xie, L., Kang, H., Xu, Q., Chen, M. J., Liao, Y., Thiyagarajan, M., ... & Takano, T. (2013). Sleep drives metabolite clearance from the adult brain. *science, 342*(6156), 373-377.

38   van Dongen, E. V., Takashima, A., Barth, M., Zapp, J., Schad, L. R., Paller, K. A., & Fernández, G. (2012). Memory stabilization with targeted reactivation during human slow-wave sleep. Proceedings of the National Academy of Sciences, 109(26), 10575-10580.

39   Saletin, J. M., & Walker, M. P. (2012). Nocturnal mnemonics: sleep and hippocampal memory processing. Frontiers in Neurology, 3.

40   Born, J., & Wilhelm, I. (2012). System consolidation of memory during sleep. Psychological research, 76(2), 192-203.

41   Zhao, Z., Zhao, X., & Veasey, S. C. (2017). Neural Consequences of Chronic Short Sleep: Reversible or Lasting?. *Frontiers in Neurology*, 8.

42   Van Dongen, H. P., Maislin, G., Mullington, J. M., & Dinges, D. F. (2003). The cumulative cost of additional wakefulness: dose-response effects on neurobehavioral functions and sleep physiology from chronic sleep restriction and total sleep deprivation. *Sleep, 26*(2), 117-126.

43   Deliens, G., Leproult, R., Neu, D., & Peigneux, P. (2013). Rapid eye movement and non-rapid eye movement sleep contributions in memory consolidation and resistance to retroactive interference for verbal material. *Sleep, 36*(12), 1875-1883.

44   Xie, L., Kang, H., Xu, Q., Chen, M. J., Liao, Y., Thiyagarajan, M., ... & Takano, T. (2013). Sleep drives metabolite clearance from the adult brain. *science, 342*(6156), 373-377.

45   Nikonova, E. V., Naidoo, N., Zhang, L., Romer, M., Cater, J. R., Scharf, M. T., ... & Pack, A. I. (2010). Changes in components of energy regulation in mouse cortex with increases in wakefulness. *Sleep, 33*(7), 889-900.

46   Van Someren EJ. Mechanisms and functions of coupling between sleep and temperature rhythms. Prog Brain Res. 2006;153: 309-24.

47   Howatson, G., Bell, P. G., Tallent, J., Middleton, B., McHugh, M. P., & Ellis, J. (2012). Effect of tart cherry juice (Prunus cerasus) on melatonin levels and enhanced sleep quality. *European journal of nutrition, 51*(8), 909-916.

48   Espino, J., Pariente, J. A., & Rodríguez, A. B. (2012). Oxidative stress and immunosenescence: therapeutic effects of melatonin. *Oxidative medicine and cellular longevity, 2012*.

49   Antony, J. W., & Paller, K. A. (2017). Using Oscillating Sounds to Manipulate Sleep Spindles. *Sleep, 40*(3).

50   Black, D. S., O'Reilly, G. A., Olmstead, R., Breen, E. C., & Irwin, M. R. (2015). Mindfulness meditation and improvement in sleep quality and daytime impairment among older adults with sleep disturbances: a randomized clinical trial. *JAMA internal medicine, 175*(4), 494-501.

51   Hölzel, B. K., Carmody, J., Vangel, M., Congleton, C., Yerramsetti, S. M., Gard,

T., & Lazar, S. W. (2011). Mindfulness practice leads to increases in regional brain gray matter density. *Psychiatry Research: Neuroimaging*, *191*(1), 36-43.

52 Westrich, L., & Sprouse, J. (2010). Circadian rhythm dysregulation in bipolar disorder. *Current opinion in investigational drugs (London, England: 2000)*, *11*(7), 779-787.

53 Ehlers, C. L., Somes, C., Seifritz, E., & Rivier, J. E. (1997). CRF/NPY interactions: a potential role in sleep dysregulation in depression and anxiety. *Depression and anxiety*, *6*(1), 1-9.

54 Li, J. Z., Bunney, B. G., Meng, F., Hagenauer, M. H., Walsh, D. M., Vawter, M. P., ... & Schatzberg, A. F. (2013). Circadian patterns of gene expression in the human brain and disruption in major depressive disorder. *Proceedings of the National Academy of Sciences*, *110*(24), 9950-9955.

55 Monti, J. M., BaHammam, A. S., Pandi-Perumal, S. R., Bromundt, V., Spence, D. W., Cardinali, D. P., & Brown, G. M. (2013). Sleep and circadian rhythm dysregulation in schizophrenia. *Progress in Neuro-Psychopharmacology and Biological Psychiatry*, *43*, 209-216.

56 Evans, J. A., & Davidson, A. J. (2013). Health consequences of circadian disruption in humans and animal models. *Prog Mol Biol Transl Sci*, *119*, 283-323.

57 Laposky, A. D., Bass, J., Kohsaka, A., & Turek, F. W. (2008). Sleep and circadian rhythms: key components in the regulation of energy metabolism. *FEBS letters*, *582*(1), 142-151.

58 Laposky, A. D., Bass, J., Kohsaka, A., & Turek, F. W. (2008). Sleep and circadian rhythms: key components in the regulation of energy metabolism. *FEBS letters*, *582*(1), 142-151.

59 Lin, J. D., Liu, C., & Li, S. (2008). Integration of energy metabolism and the mammalian clock. *Cell Cycle*, *7*(4), 453-457.

60 Morris, M. C., Evans, D. A., Bienias, J. L., Tangney, C. C., & Wilson, R. S. (2004). Dietary fat intake and 6-year cognitive change in an o

61 Barnard, N. D., Bush, A. I., Ceccarelli, A., Cooper, J., de Jager, C. A., Erickson, K. I., ... & Morris, M. C. (2014). Dietary and lifestyle guidelines for the prevention of Alzheimer's disease. *Neurobiology of Aging*, *35*, S74-S78.

62 Golomb BA, Bui AK (2015) A Fat to Forget: Trans Fat Consumption and Memory. PLoS ONE 10(6): e0128129. https://doi.org/10.1371/journal.pone.0128129

63 Sánchez-Villegas, A., Verberne, L., De Irala, J., Ruíz-Canela, M., Toledo, E., Serra-Majem, L., & Martínez-González, M. A. (2011). Dietary fat intake and the risk of depression: the SUN Project. *PloS one*, *6*(1), e16268.

64 Yeomans, M. R. (2017). Adverse effects of consuming high fat–sugar diets on cognition: implications for understanding obesity. *Proceedings of the Nutrition Society*, 1-11.

65 Beilharz, J. E., Maniam, J., & Morris, M. J. (2015). Diet-induced cognitive deficits: the role of fat and sugar, potential mechanisms and nutritional interventions. *Nutrients*, *7*(8), 6719-6738.

66 Lakhan, S. E., & Kirchgessner, A. (2013). The emerging role of dietary fructose in obesity and cognitive decline. *Nutr J*, *12*(1), 114-25.

67 Strachan, M. W. J. (2005). Insulin and cognitive function in humans: experimental data and therapeutic considerations.

68 Domínguez, R., Cuenca, E., Maté-Muñoz, J. L., García-Fernández, P., Serra-Paya, N., Estevan, M. C. L., ... & Garnacho-Castaño, M. V. (2017). Effects of Beetroot Juice Supplementation on Cardiorespiratory Endurance in Athletes. A Systematic Review. *Nutrients*, *9*(1), 43.

69   Curry, B. H., Bond, V., Pemminati, S., Gorantla, V. R., Volkova, Y. A., Kadur, K., & Millis, R. M. (2016). Effects of a Dietary Beetroot Juice Treatment on Systemic and Cerebral Haemodynamics–A Pilot Study. *Journal of clinical and diagnostic research: JCDR*, *10*(7), CC01.

70   Haskell-Ramsay, C. F., Stuart, R. C., Okello, E. J., & Watson, A. W. (2017). Cognitive and mood improvements following acute supplementation with purple grape juice in healthy young adults. *European Journal of Nutrition*, 1-11.

71   Georgiev, V., Ananga, A., & Tsolova, V. (2014). Recent advances and uses of grape flavonoids as nutraceuticals. *Nutrients*, *6*(1), 391-415.

72   Chen, N., Yang, M., Zhou, M., Xiao, J., Guo, J., & He, L. (2017). L-carnitine for cognitive enhancement in people without cognitive impairment. *The Cochrane Library*.

73   Rawson, E. S., Lieberman, H. R., Walsh, T. M., Zuber, S. M., Harhart, J. M., & Matthews, T. C. (2008). Creatine supplementation does not improve cognitive function in young adults. *Physiology & behavior*, *95*(1), 130-134.

74   Owen, L., & Sunram-Lea, S. I. (2011). Metabolic agents that enhance ATP can improve cognitive functioning: a review of the evidence for glucose, oxygen, pyruvate, creatine, and L-carnitine. *Nutrients*, *3*(8), 735-755.

75   Sullivan, P. G., Geiger, J. D., Mattson, M. P., & Scheff, S. W. (2000). Dietary supplement creatine protects against traumatic brain injury. *Annals of neurology*, *48*(5), 723-729.

76   Ling, J., Kritikos, M., & Tiplady, B. (2009). Cognitive effects of creatine ethyl ester supplementation. *Behavioural pharmacology*, *20*(8), 673-679.

77   McMorris, T., Harris, R. C., Swain, J., Corbett, J., Collard, K., Dyson, R. J., ... & Draper, N. (2006). Effect of creatine supplementation and sleep deprivation, with mild exercise, on cognitive and psychomotor performance, mood state, and plasma concentrations of catecholamines and cortisol. *Psychopharmacology*, *185*(1), 93-103.

78   Yoshikawa, T., Nakamura, T., Shibakusa, T., Sugita, M., Naganuma, F., Iida, T., ... & Yanai, K. (2014). Insufficient intake of L-histidine reduces brain histamine and causes anxiety-like behaviors in male mice. *The Journal of nutrition*, *144*(10), 1637-1641.

79   Grams, L., Garrido, G., Villacieros, J., & Ferro, A. (2016). Marginal Micronutrient Intake in High-Performance Male Wheelchair Basketball Players: A Dietary Evaluation and the Effects of Nutritional Advice. *PloS one*, *11*(7), e0157931.

80   Table, E., & Table, V. (2001). Dietary reference intakes for vitamin A, vitamin K, arsenic, boron, chromium, copper, iodine, iron, manganese, molybdenum, nickel, silicon, vanadium, and zinc.

81   Wenger, M. J., DellaValle, D. M., Murray-Kolb, L. E., & Haas, J. D. (2017). Effect of iron deficiency on simultaneous measures of behavior, brain activity, and energy expenditure in the performance of a cognitive task. *Nutritional neuroscience*, 1-10.

82   Kuszewski, J. C., Wong, R. H., & Howe, P. R. (2017). Effects of Long-Chain Omega-3 Polyunsaturated Fatty Acids on Endothelial Vasodilator Function and Cognition—Are They Interrelated? *Nutrients*, *9*(5), 487.

83   Packer, L., & Cadenas, E. (2010). Lipoic acid: energy metabolism and redox regulation of transcription and cell signaling. *Journal of clinical biochemistry and nutrition*, *48*(1), 26-32.

84   Gillberg, I.C., Billstedt, E., Wentz, E., Anckarsater, H., Rastam, M., & Gillberg, C. (2010). Attention, executive functions, and mentalizing in anorexia nervosa eighteen years after onset of eating disorder. In Journal of Clinical and Experimental Neuropsychology (Vol. 32, Issue 4).

85   Williams, J., & Taylor, E. (2004). Dopamine appetite and cognitive impairment in attention deficit/hyperactivity disorder. Neural plasticity, 11(1-2), 115-132.

86   Biederman, J., Monuteaux, M. C., Doyle, A. E., Seidman, L. J., Wilens, T. E., Ferrero, F., ... & Faraone, S. V. (2004). Impact of executive function deficits and attention-deficit/hyperactivity disorder (ADHD) on academic outcomes in children. *Journal of consulting and clinical psychology, 72*(5), 757.

87   Bond, A. J. (2001). Neurotransmitters, temperament and social functioning. European Neuropsychopharmacology, 11(4), 261-274.

88   Bates, J. E., & Wachs, T. D. (1994). Temperament: Individual differences at the interface of biology and behavior. American Psychological Association.

89   Rueda, M. R., Posner, M. I., & Rothbart, M. K. (2005). The development of executive attention: Contributions to the emergence of self-regulation. Developmental neuropsychology, 28(2), 573-594.

90   Rothbart, M. K., & Posner, M. I. (2005). Genes and experience in the development of executive attention and effortful control. New Directions for Child and Adolescent Development, 2005(109), 101-108.

91   Posner, M. I., & Rothbart, M. K. (2000). Developing mechanisms of self-regulation. Development and Psychopathology, 12, 427-441

92   Rothbart, M. K., Ahadi, S. A., & Evans, D. E. (2000). Temperament and personality: origins and outcomes. Journal of personality and social psychology, 78(1), 122.

93   Thakkar, M. M. (2011). Histamine in the regulation of wakefulness. Sleep medicine reviews, 15(1), 65-74.

94   Le, S., Gruner, J. A., Mathiasen, J. R., Marino, M. J., & Schaffhauser, H. (2008). Correlation between ex vivo receptor occupancy and wake-promoting activity of selective H3 receptor antagonists. Journal of Pharmacology and Experimental Therapeutics, 325(3), 902-909.

95   Broderick, M., & Guilleminault, C. (2016). Emerging treatments for narcolepsy. In Narcolepsy (pp. 357-368). Springer International Publishing.

96   Abbott, N. J. (2000). Inflammatory mediators and modulation of blood–brain barrier permeability. Cellular and molecular neurobiology, 20(2), 131-147.

97   Maintz, L., & Novak, N. (2007). Histamine and histamine intolerance. The American journal of clinical nutrition, 85(5), 1185-1196.

98   Vally, Hassan, and PHILIP THOMPSON. "Allergic and asthmatic reactions to alcoholic drinks." Addiction biology 8.1 (2003): 3-11.

99   Sattler, J., Hesterberg, R., Schmidt, U., Crombach, M., & Lorenz, W. (1987). Inhibition of intestinal diamine oxidase by detergents: a problem for drug formulations with water insoluble agents applied by the intravenous route?. Inflammation Research, 20(3), 270-273.

100 Tsujino, N., & Sakurai, T. (2009). Orexin/hypocretin: a neuropeptide at the interface of sleep, energy homeostasis, and reward system. Pharmacological reviews, 61(2), 162-176.

101 Tsujino, N., Yamanaka, A., Ichiki, K., Muraki, Y., Kilduff, T. S., Yagami, K. I., ... & Sakurai, T. (2005). Cholecystokinin activates orexin/hypocretin neurons through the cholecystokinin A receptor. Journal of Neuroscience, 25(32), 7459-7469.

102 Brown, R. E., Basheer, R., McKenna, J. T., Strecker, R. E., & McCarley, R. W. (2012). Control of sleep and wakefulness. *Physiological reviews, 92*(3), 1087-1187.

103   Young, S. N. (2007). How to increase serotonin in the human brain without drugs. *Journal of psychiatry & neuroscience: JPN*,*32*(6), 394.

104   Drevets, W. C., Thase, M. E., Moses-Kolko, E. L., Price, J., Frank, E., Kupfer, D. J., & Mathis, C. (2007). Serotonin-1A receptor imaging in recurrent depression: replication and literature review. *Nuclear medicine and biology*, *34*(7), 865-877.

105   Shim, R. S., Baltrus, P., Ye, J., & Rust, G. (2011). Prevalence, treatment, and control of depressive symptoms in the United States: results from the National Health and Nutrition Examination Survey (NHANES), 2005–2008. *The Journal of the American Board of Family Medicine*, *24*(1), 33-38.

106   Gryglewski, G., Lanzenberger, R., Kranz, G. S., & Cumming, P. (2014). Meta-analysis of molecular imaging of serotonin transporters in major depression. *Journal of Cerebral Blood Flow & Metabolism*, *34*(7), 1096-1103.

107   Sansone, R. A., & Sansone, L. A. (2013). Sunshine, serotonin, and skin: a partial explanation for seasonal patterns in psychopathology?. Innovations in clinical neuroscience, 10(7-8), 20.

108   Brown, R. E., Basheer, R., McKenna, J. T., Strecker, R. E., & McCarley, R. W. (2012). Control of sleep and wakefulness. *Physiological reviews*, *92*(3), 1087-1187.

109   Knab, A. M., & Lightfoot, J. T. (2010). Does the difference between physically active and couch potato lie in the dopamine system? *International journal of biological sciences*, *6*(2), 133.

110   Kjaer, T. W., Bertelsen, C., Piccini, P., Brooks, D., Alving, J., & Lou, H. C. (2002). Increased dopamine tone during meditation-induced change of consciousness. *Cognitive Brain Research*, *13*(2), 255-259.

111   Aston-Jones, G., & Cohen, J. D. (2005). An integrative theory of locus coeruleus-norepinephrine function: adaptive gain and optimal performance. *Annu. Rev. Neurosci.*, *28*, 403-450.

112   Xing, B., Li, Y. C., & Gao, W. J. (2016). Norepinephrine versus dopamine and their interaction in modulating synaptic function in the prefrontal cortex. *brain research*, *1641*, 217-233.

113   Crum, A. J., Salovey, P., & Achor, S. (2013). Rethinking stress: The role of mindsets in determining the stress response. *Journal of personality and social psychology*, *104*(4), 716.

114   Jamieson, J. P., Nock, M. K., & Mendes, W. B. (2012). Mind over matter: Reappraising arousal improves cardiovascular and cognitive responses to stress. Journal of Experimental Psychology: General, 141(3), 417.

115   Keller, A., Litzelman, K., Wisk, L. E., Maddox, T., Cheng, E. R., Creswell, P. D., & Witt, W. P. (2012). Does the perception that stress affects health matter? The association with health and mortality. Health Psychology, 31(5), 677.

116   Cahill, L., & Alkire, M. T. (2003). Epinephrine enhancement of human memory consolidation: interaction with arousal at encoding. *Neurobiology of learning and memory*, *79*(2), 194-198.

117   Gold, P. E. (2014). Regulation of memory–From the adrenal medulla to liver to astrocytes to neurons. *Brain research bulletin*, *105*, 25-35.

118   Xing, B., Li, Y. C., & Gao, W. J. (2016). Norepinephrine versus dopamine and their interaction in modulating synaptic function in the prefrontal cortex. *brain research*, *1641*, 217-233.

119   Gomez-Pinilla, F., & Hillman, C. (2013). The influence of exercise on cognitive

abilities. Comprehensive Physiology.

120   Vaynman, S., Ying, Z., & Gomez-Pinilla, F. (2004). Hippocampal BDNF mediates the efficacy of exercise on synaptic plasticity and cognition. European Journal of Neuroscience, 20(10), 2580-2590.

121   Sleiman, S. F., Henry, J., Al-Haddad, R., El Hayek, L., Haidar, E. A., Stringer, T., ... & Ninan, I. (2016). Exercise promotes the expression of brain derived neurotrophic factor (BDNF) through the action of the ketone body β-hydroxybutyrate. Elife, 5, e15092.

122   Oztasyonar, Y. (2017). Interaction between different sports branches such as taekwondo, box, athletes and serum brain derived neurotrophic factor levels. The Journal of sports medicine and physical fitness, 57(4), 457-460.

123   Heydari, G. R., Ramezankhani, A., & Talischi, F. (2011). The impacts of cigarette packaging pictorial warning labels on smokers in the city of Tehran. Tanaffos, 10(1), 40.

124   Gomez-Pinilla, F., & Hillman, C. (2013). The influence of exercise on cognitive abilities. Comprehensive Physiology.

125   Oztasyonar, Y. (2017). Interaction between different sports branches such as taekwondo, box, athletes and serum brain derived neurotrophic factor levels. *The Journal of sports medicine and physical fitness*, 57(4), 457-460.

126   Douris, P., Douris, C., Balder, N., LaCasse, M., Rand, A., Tarapore, F., ... & Handrakis, J. (2015). Martial art training and cognitive performance in middle-aged adults. Journal of human kinetics, 47(1), 277-283.

127   Borghouts, L. B., & Keizer, H. A. (2000). Exercise and insulin sensitivity: a review. International journal of sports medicine, 21(01), 1-12.

128   Randolph, D. D., & O'Connor, P. J. (2017). Stair walking is more energizing than low dose caffeine in sleep deprived young women. Physiology & Behavior, 174, 128-135.

129   Perello, M., & Dickson, S. L. (2015). Ghrelin signalling on food reward: a salient link between the gut and the mesolimbic system. Journal of neuroendocrinology, 27(6), 424-434.

130   Di Chiara, G., & Bassareo, V. (2007). Reward system and addiction: what dopamine does and doesn't do. Current opinion in pharmacology, 7(1), 69-76.

131   Pico, C., Oliver, P., Sanchez, J., & Palou, A. (2003). Gastric leptin: a putative role in the short-term regulation of food intake. British Journal of Nutrition, 90(4), 735-741.

132   Colldén, G., Tschöp, M. H., & Müller, T. D. (2017). Therapeutic Potential of Targeting the Ghrelin Pathway. International journal of molecular sciences, 18(4), 798.

133   Meyer, R. M., Burgos-Robles, A., Liu, E., Correia, S. S., & Goosens, K. A. (2014). A ghrelin–growth hormone axis drives stress-induced vulnerability to enhanced fear. Molecular psychiatry, 19(12), 1284-1294.

134   Portelli, J., Thielemans, L., Ver Donck, L., Loyens, E., Coppens, J., Aourz, N., ... & Michotte, Y. (2012). Inactivation of the constitutively active ghrelin receptor attenuates limbic seizure activity in rodents. Neurotherapeutics, 9(3), 658-672.

135   Franke, A. G., Gränsmark, P., Agricola, A., Schuehle, K., Rommel, T., Sebastian, A., ... & Ruckes, C. (2017). Methylphenidate, modafinil, and caffeine for cognitive enhancement in chess: A double-blind, randomized controlled trial. European Neuropsychopharmacology, 27(3), 248-260.

136   De Pauw, K., Roelands, B., Knaepen, K., Polfliet, M., Stiens, J., & Meeusen, R. (2015). Effects of caffeine and maltodextrin mouth rinsing on P300, brain imaging, and cognitive performance. Journal of Applied Physiology, 118(6), 776-782.

137   Juneja, L. R., Chu, D. C., Okubo, T., Nagato, Y., & Yokogoshi, H. (1999). L-theanine—a unique amino acid of green tea and its relaxation effect in humans. *Trends in Food Science & Technology, 10*(6-7), 199-204.

138   Vidyasagar, R., Greyling, A., Draijer, R., Corfield, D. R., & Parkes, L. M. (2013). The effect of black tea and caffeine on regional cerebral blood flow measured with arterial spin labeling. *Journal of Cerebral Blood Flow & Metabolism, 33*(6), 963-968.

139   Chang, C. W., Wang, S. H., Jan, M. Y., & Wang, W. K. (2017). Effect of black tea consumption on radial blood pulse spectrum and cognitive health. *Complementary Therapies in Medicine, 31*, 1-7.

140   Dodd, F. L., Kennedy, D. O., Riby, L. M., & Haskell-Ramsay, C. F. (2015). A double-blind, placebo-controlled study evaluating the effects of caffeine and L-theanine both alone and in combination on cerebral blood flow, cognition and mood. *Psychopharmacology, 232*(14), 2563-2576.

141   Rogers, P. J., Smith, J. E., Heatherley, S. V., & Pleydell-Pearce, C. W. (2008). Time for tea: mood, blood pressure and cognitive performance effects of caffeine and theanine administered alone and together. *Psychopharmacology, 195*(4), 569.

142   Owen, G. N., Parnell, H., De Bruin, E. A., & Rycroft, J. A. (2008). The combined effects of L-theanine and caffeine on cognitive performance and mood. *Nutritional neuroscience, 11*(4), 193-198.

143   Dietz, C., & Dekker, M. (2017). Effect of Green Tea Phytochemicals on Mood and Cognition. *Current pharmaceutical design*.

144   Colosio, M., Shestakova, A., Nikulin, V. V., Blagovechtchenski, E., & Klucharev, V. (2017). Neural mechanisms of cognitive dissonance (revised): An EEG study. *Journal of Neuroscience, 37*(20), 5074-5083.

145   Baumeister, R. F., Stillwell, A. M., & Heatherton, T. F. (1994). Guilt: an interpersonal approach. *Psychological bulletin, 115*(2), 243.

146   Crespo-Bojorque, P., & Toro, J. M. (2016). Processing advantages for consonance: A comparison between rats (Rattus norvegicus) and humans (Homo sapiens). *Journal of Comparative Psychology, 130*(2), 97.

147   Kurtz, J. L., & Lyubomirsky, S. (2008). Towards a durable happiness. The positive psychology perspective series, 4, 21-36.

148   Sheldon, K. M., & Lyubomirsky, S. (2006). Achieving sustainable gains in happiness: Change your actions, not your circumstances. Journal of Happiness Studies, 7(1), 55-86.

149   Farhud, D. D., Malmir, M., & Khanahmadi, M. (2014). Happiness & Health: The Biological Factors-Systematic Review Article. Iranian Journal of Public Health, 43(11).

150   McCullough, M. E., & Emmons, R. A. (2003). Counting blessings versus burdens: an experimental investigation of gratitude and subjective well-being in daily life. J. Pers. Soc. Psychol., 84, 377-389.

151   Disabato, D. J., Kashdan, T. B., Short, J. L., & Jarden, A. (2017). What predicts positive life events that influence the course of depression? A longitudinal examination of gratitude and meaning in life. Cognitive Therapy and Research, 41(3), 444-458.

152   Wild, B., Erb, M., & Bartels, M. (2001). Are emotions contagious? Evoked emotions while viewing emotionally expressive faces: quality, quantity, time course and gender differences. Psychiatry research, 102(2), 109-124.

153   Wagner, U., Galli, L., Schott, B. H., Wold, A., van der Schalk, J., Manstead, A. S., ... & Walter, H. (2014). Beautiful friendship: social sharing of emotions improves subjective feelings and activates the neural reward circuitry. Social cognitive and affective neuroscience,

10(6), 801-808.

154	Nummenmaa, L., Glerean, E., Viinikainen, M., Jääskeläinen, I. P., Hari, R., & Sams, M. (2012). Emotions promote social interaction by synchronizing brain activity across individuals. Proceedings of the National Academy of Sciences, 109(24), 9599-9604.

155	Zautra, A. J., Affleck, G. G., Tennen, H., Reich, J. W., & Davis, M. C. (2005). Dynamic approaches to emotions and stress in everyday life: Bolger and Zuckerman reloaded with positive as well as negative affects. Journal of personality, 73(6), 1511-1538.

156	Musick, M. A., & Wilson, J. (2003). Volunteering and depression: The role of psychological and social resources in different age groups. Social science & medicine, 56(2), 259-269.

157	Crockett, M. J. (2009). The neurochemistry of fairness: clarifying the link between serotonin and prosocial behavior. Annals of the New York Academy of Sciences, 1167(1), 76-86.

158	Mehl, M. R., Vazire, S., Holleran, S. E., & Clark, C. S. (2010). Eavesdropping on happiness: Well-being is related to having less small talk and more substantive conversations. Psychological science, 21(4), 539-541.

159	Tversky, A., & Kahneman, D. (1991). Loss aversion in riskless choice: A reference-dependent model. The quarterly journal of economics, 106(4), 1039-1061.

160	Brickman, P., Coates, D., & Janoff-Bulman, R. (1978). Lottery winners and accident victims: Is happiness relative?. Journal of personality and social psychology, 36(8), 917.

161	Starcke, K., Agorku, J. D., & Brand, M. (2017). Exposure to Unsolvable Anagrams Impairs Performance on the Iowa Gambling Task. *Frontiers in Behavioral Neuroscience*, 11, 114.

162	Miller, W. R., & Seligman, M. E. (1975). Depression and learned helplessness in man. *Journal of abnormal psychology*, 84(3), 228.

163	Gregg, M. J., & Clark, T. (2007). Theoretical and practical applications of mental imagery. In *Proceedings of the International Symposium on Performance Science* (pp. 295-300).

164	Sheridan, H., & Reingold, E. M. (2014). Expert vs. novice differences in the detection of relevant information during a chess game: evidence from eye movements. Frontiers in psychology, 5, 941.

165	Marsh, J. E., & Campbell, T. A. (2016). Processing complex sounds passing through the rostral brainstem: The new early filter model. *Frontiers in neuroscience*, 10.

166	Raichle, M. E., & Gusnard, D. A. (2002). Appraising the brain's energy budget. *Proceedings of the National Academy of Sciences*, 99(16), 10237-10239.

167	Sibson, N. R., Dhankhar, A., Mason, G. F., Rothman, D. L., Behar, K. L., & Shulman, R. G. (1998). Stoichiometric coupling of brain glucose metabolism and glutamatergic neuronal activity. *Proceedings of the National Academy of Sciences*, 95(1), 316-321.

168	Theeuwes, J. (1991). Exogenous and endogenous control of attention: The effect of visual onsets and offsets. *Attention, Perception, & Psychophysics*, 49(1), 83-90.

169	Hameed, S., Ferris, T., Jayaraman, S., & Sarter, N. (2009). Using informative peripheral visual and tactile cues to support task and interruption management. *Human factors*, 51(2), 126-135.

170	Marsh, J. E., Ljung, R., Nöstl, A., Threadgold, E., & Campbell, T. A. (2015). Failing to get the gist of what's being said: background noise impairs higher-order cognitive processing. *Frontiers in psychology*, 6.

171	Mak, C. M., & Lui, Y. P. (2012). The effect of sound on office productivity. *Building Services Engineering Research and Technology*, 33(3), 339-345.

172 Hartley, James, & Davies, Ivor K. (1986). Note-taking: A critical review. *Programmed Learning and Educational Technology*, 15, 207.

173 Corbetta, M, Patel, G, & Shulman, GL. (2008). The reorienting system of the human brain: from environment to theory of mind. Neuron, 58(3), 306-324.

174 Baumeister, Roy F, Bratslavsky, Ellen, Muraven, Mark, & Tice, Dianne M. (1998). Ego depletion: Is the active self a limited resource? *Journal of Personality and Social Psychology*, 74(5), 1252-1265.

175 Houghton, G. (1996). Inhibition and interference in selective attention: Some tests of a neural network model. Visual Cognition, 3(2), 119-164.

176 Kuhl, Brice A, Kahn, Itamar, Dudukovic, Nicole M, & Wagner, Anthony D. (2008). Overcoming suppression in order to remember: Contributions from anterior cingulate and ventrolateral prefrontal cortex. Cognitive Affective & Behavioral Neuroscience, 8(2), 211-221.

177 Lieberman, Matthew D. (2009). The brain's braking system (and how to 'use your words' to tap into it). NeuroLeadership Journal, 2, 9-14.

178 Marsh, J. E., & Campbell, T. A. (2016). Processing complex sounds passing through the rostral brainstem: The new early filter model. Frontiers in neuroscience, 10.

179 Morita, K., Morishima, M., Sakai, K., & Kawaguchi, Y. (2013). Dopaminergic control of motivation and reinforcement learning: a closed-circuit account for reward-oriented behavior. *Journal of Neuroscience*, 33(20), 8866-8890.

180 Schultheiss, O. C., & Wirth, M. M. (2008). Biopsychological aspects of motivation.

181 Fernández-Lamo, I., Delgado-García, J. M., & Gruart, A. (2017). When and Where Learning is Taking Place: Multisynaptic Changes in Strength During Different Behaviors Related to the Acquisition of an Operant Conditioning Task by Behaving Rats. *Cerebral Cortex*, 1-13.

182 Tompson, S., Lieberman, M. D., & Falk, E. B. (2015). Grounding the neuroscience of behavior change in the sociocultural context. *Current Opinion in Behavioral Sciences*, 5, 58-63.

183 Hecht, D. (2013). The neural basis of optimism and pessimism. *Experimental neurobiology*, 22(3), 173-199.

184 Alvarez, J., Day, D., Gardner, A., Saeed, I., Schwebach, C., & Valk, R. (2015). Effectiveness of Stress Balls in Reducing the Physiological Symptoms of Stress.

185 Hiroto, D. S., & Seligman, M. E. (1975). Generality of learned helplessness in man. *Journal of personality and social psychology*, 31(2), 311.

186 Mark, G., Gudith, D., & Klocke, U. (2008, April). The cost of interrupted work: more speed and stress. In Proceedings of the SIGCHI conference on Human Factors in Computing Systems (pp. 107-110). ACM.

187 Millward, D. J., Garlick, P. J., Stewart, R. J., Nnanyelugo, D. O., & Waterlow, J. C. (1975). Skeletal-muscle growth and protein turnover. Biochemical Journal, 150(2), 235-243.

188 Maquet, P. (2001). The role of sleep in learning and memory. science, 294(5544), 1048-1052.

189 Cohen, D., Cohen, M., & Cross, H. (1981). A construct validity study of the Myers-Briggs Type Indicator. Educational and Psychological Measurement, 41(3), 883-891.

190 Wu, Y., Johnson, B. T., Acabchuk, R. L., Chen, S., Lewis, H. K., Livingston, J., ... & Pescatello, L. S. (2019, March). Yoga as antihypertensive lifestyle therapy: a systematic review and meta-analysis. In Mayo Clinic Proceedings (Vol. 94, No. 3, pp. 432-446). Elsevier.

191   Kiecolt-Glaser, J. K., Christian, L., Preston, H., Houts, C. R., Malarkey, W. B., Emery, C. F., & Glaser, R. (2010). Stress, inflammation, and yoga practice. Psychosomatic medicine, 72(2), 113.

192   Cramer, H., Lauche, R., Anheyer, D., Pilkington, K., de Manincor, M., Dobos, G., & Ward, L. (2018). Yoga for anxiety: A systematic review and meta-analysis of randomized controlled trials. Depression and anxiety, 35(9), 830-843.

193   Paganoni, S. (2018). Evidence-Based Physiatry: Clinical Practice Guideline Noninvasive Treatments for Low Back Pain. American journal of physical medicine & rehabilitation, 97(10), 763.

194   Skelly, A. C., Chou, R., Dettori, J. R., Turner, J. A., Friedly, J. L., Rundell, S. D., ... & Ferguson, A. J. (2018). Noninvasive nonpharmacological treatment for chronic pain: a systematic review.

195   Kanaya, A. M., Araneta, M. R. G., Pawlowsky, S. B., Barrett-Connor, E., Grady, D., Vittinghoff, E., ... & Tanori, D. (2014). Restorative yoga and metabolic risk factors: the Practicing Restorative Yoga vs. Stretching for the Metabolic Syndrome (PRYSMS) randomized trial. Journal of Diabetes and its Complications, 28(3), 406-412.

196   Kabat-Zinn, J., & Hanh, T. N. (2009). Full catastrophe living: Using the wisdom of your body and mind to face stress, pain, and illness. Delta.

197   Hildebrandt, L. K., McCall, C., & Singer, T. (2017). Differential effects of attention-, compassion-, and socio-cognitively based mental practices on self-reports of mindfulness and compassion. Mindfulness, 8(6), 1488-1512.

198   Barnhofer, T., & Germer, C. (2017). Mindfulness and compassion: similarities and differences. In Compassion (pp. 81-98). Routledge.

199   Desbordes, G., Gard, T., Hoge, E. A., Hölzel, B. K., Kerr, C., Lazar, S. W., ... & Vago, D. R. (2015). Moving beyond mindfulness: defining equanimity as an outcome measure in meditation and contemplative research. Mindfulness, 6(2), 356-372.

200   Hofmann, S. G., Grossman, P., & Hinton, D. E. (2011). Loving-kindness and compassion meditation: Potential for psychological interventions. Clinical psychology review, 31(7), 1126-1132.

201   Chiarello, C., Burgess, C., Richards, L., & Pollock, A. (1990). Semantic and associative priming in the cerebral hemispheres: Some words do, some words don't... sometimes, some places. Brain and language, 38(1), 75-104.

202   Stanovich, K. E., & West, R. F. (1983). On priming by a sentence context. Journal of experimental psychology: General, 112(1), 1.

203   Brainerd, C. J., Yang, Y., Reyna, V. F., Howe, M. L., & Mills, B. A. (2008). Semantic processing in "associative" false memory. Psychonomic Bulletin & Review, 15(6), 1035-1053.

204   Carlson, M., Charlin, V., & Miller, N. (1988). Positive mood and helping behavior: A test of six hypotheses. Journal of personality and social psychology, 55(2), 211.

205   Erisman, S. M., & Roemer, L. (2010). A preliminary investigation of the effects of experimentally induced mindfulness on emotional responding to film clips. Emotion, 10, 72–82.

206   MacLeod, A. K., & Conway, C. (2005). Well-being and the anticipation of future positive experiences: The role of income, social networks, and planning ability. Cognition and Emotion, 19, 357–373.

207   Quoidbach, J., Wood, A., & Hansenne, M. (2009). Back to the future: The effect of daily practice of mental time travel into the future on happiness and anxiety. The Journal of Positive Psychology, 4, 349–355.

208   Ellison, C. G., & Fan, D. (2008). Daily spiritual experiences and psychological well-being among US adults. Social Indicators Research, 88(2), 247-271.

209   Weinstein, N., & Ryan, R. M. (2010). When helping helps: autonomous motivation for prosocial behavior and its influence on well-being for the helper and recipient. Journal of personality and social psychology, 98(2), 222.

210   Bernardi, L., Sleight, P., Bandinelli, G., Cencetti, S., Fattorini, L., Wdowczyc-Szulc, J., & Lagi, A. (2001). Effect of rosary prayer and yoga mantras on autonomic cardiovascular rhythms: comparative study. Bmj, 323(7327), 1446-1449.

211   Goessl, V. C., Curtiss, J. E., & Hofmann, S. G. (2017). The effect of heart rate variability biofeedback training on stress and anxiety: a meta-analysis. Psychological medicine, 47(15), 2578-2586.

212   Zelano, C., Jiang, H., Zhou, G., Arora, N., Schuele, S., Rosenow, J., & Gottfried, J. A. (2016). Nasal respiration entrains human limbic oscillations and modulates cognitive function. Journal of Neuroscience, 36(49), 12448-12467.

213   Ochsner, K. N., Silvers, J. A., & Buhle, J. T. (2012). Functional imaging studies of emotion regulation: a synthetic review and evolving model of the cognitive control of emotion. Annals of the New York Academy of Sciences, 1251(1), E1-E24.

214   Krishnakumar, D., Hamblin, M. R., & Lakshmanan, S. (2015). Meditation and yoga can modulate brain mechanisms that affect behavior and anxiety-A modern scientific perspective. Ancient science, 2(1), 13.

215   Guglietti, C. L., Daskalakis, Z. J., Radhu, N., Fitzgerald, P. B., & Ritvo, P. (2013). Meditation-related increases in GABAB modulated cortical inhibition. Brain stimulation, 6(3), 397-402.

216   Trappe, H. J. (2012). Music and medicine: The effects of music on the human being. Applied Cardiopulmonary Pathophysiology, 16(1), 133-142.

217   Trappe, H. J. (2010). The effects of music on the cardiovascular system and cardiovascular health. Heart, 96(23), 1868-1871.

Index

80/20 170

Adrenaline 97, 98, 100

alcohol 14, 30, 37, 57

almonds 42, 68

Amino acids 11, 92

AMPK 25, 26, 104, 106

amygdala 92, 96, 103, 105, 108, 129

anthocyanin 59

anti-inflammatory 59, 60

ATP 16, 17, 23, 24, 25, 36, 40, 61, 62, 70, 73, 205

auditory cortex 155, 156

avocados 53, 54, 68

Baumeister, Roy 129

beetroot 58

Belavtseva, Nadezhda 141

Beliefs 122, 147

binaural beats 42, 43

Bioenergetics 2, 5, 9

blood brain barrier 19, 20, 25, 39, 41, 62, 64, 70, 78, 97

body temperature 28, 41, 48

brain-derived neurotrophic factor 102

brain waves 43, 48

burnout 117, 118, 119, 128, 136, 138, 138–222, 175

carbohydrates 11, 54, 56, 70, 92, 106

Cerebral Blood Flow 31, 203, 207, 209

Circadian Rhythm 44, 48, 50, 159, 204

CO2 21, 22

Coaching 82

cocktail party effect 155

Coffee 15, 109, 201

Cognitive Consonance 125, 126, 127, 130, 146, 147

cognitive dissonance 126, 127, 128, 129, 209

cognitive performance 33, 37, 38, 53, 61, 66, 68, 101, 106, 111, 112, 140, 202, 208, 209

Complex Movement Cardio 104

Concentration 150

Creatine 61, 205

DARPA 114

dehydration 28, 29, 31

depression 48, 54, 92, 140, 175, 204, 207

Diamine Oxidase 79

dietary histamine 64, 78, 79, 80

Dopamine 95, 206

Drills 160

Edwards, Owen 83, 162

endothelium 58

fat 10, 13, 18, 53, 54, 56, 68, 69, 70, 204

fenugreek 42

Flavonoids 59

Florida State University 129

flow 21, 24, 28, 30, 32, 33, 34, 58, 59, 67, 70, 106, 112, 114, 150, 166, 168, 209

Freidrikson, Barbara 133

Fructose 55

GABA 79, 81

Ghrelin 81, 107, 108, 208

glucagon 201

gluconeogenesis 48

Glucose 10, 11, 12, 13, 14, 16, 17, 19, 21, 23, 24, 25, 28, 30, 34, 36, 48, 55, 59, 68, 70, 81, 98, 100, 102, 106, 108, 113, 201, 205, 210

Goals 122, 147

goji berries 42

Gokan De Ajiwau 152

grape 58, 59

green leafy vegetables 66

high-intensity interval training 26

Histamine 77, 78, 79, 81, 206

homeostasis 41, 65, 81, 105, 107, 206

Hydration 27, 202

hypoxia 26

Immersion 153, 190

insulin sensitivity 48, 69, 106, 201, 208

International Chess Federation 112

Iodine 64, 65

iron 66, 205

jogging 107

L-carnitine 61, 205

learned helplessness 140, 172, 176, 210, 211

left brain 172, 176

Leon Festinger 126
L-histidine 63, 64, 78, 79, 80, 115, 205
lipolysis 48
liver 13, 14, 15, 16, 23, 30, 55, 57, 61, 68, 70, 98, 201, 207
Locus of Control 139, 140, 148, 171, 176, 177, 178
L-Theanine 112, 113, 209
L-Tyrosine 63
Maslow, Abraham 119, 147, 148
Max Plank Institute 127
medial orbitofrontal gyrus 129
Melatonin 41
midbrain reticular formation 156
military 95, 114, 159, 160, 161, 171
Mindfulness 150, 151, 152, 168, 176, 203, 204
MIT 108
mitochondria 16, 17, 18, 23, 25, 26, 36, 38, 68, 70, 201
Mitochondrial Biogenesis 25, 26, 27, 50, 104, 202
Modafinil 114
monounsaturated fats 53
Motivation 19, 76, 95, 104, 106, 113, 115, 117, 118, 122, 125, 131, 139, 141, 148, 172, 211
mustard seeds 42
N3 Sleep 34
Negative Thinking 171, 175
neurodegenerative illnesses 60
neurosteroids 99
neurotoxins 38, 39, 70, 111

neurotransmitters 11, 64, 70, 77, 78, 79, 80, 84, 115

Noradrenaline 97, 101

olive oil 53, 54

omega-3 fatty acids 32, 67

Orexin 80, 81, 82, 206

oxygen 9, 11, 21, 22, 24, 26, 27, 28, 30, 33, 35, 36, 58, 62, 66, 70, 98, 99, 113, 201, 205

P3 wave 105

pancreas 13, 14, 15, 70

Pavio, Allan 143

PFC 33, 82, 95, 98, 101, 103, 105, 112, 127, 128, 151, 153, 155, 164, 168, 172, 174

PGC-1α 25, 26, 202

Phelps, Michael 142

pineal gland 42

Pink Noise 158

Positive Psychology 131

posterior medial frontal cortex 127

poultry 64, 66

PTSD 108

Rapid Eye Movement (REM) sleep 35

Red meat 66

ROS 36

rostrum brainstem 153, 156, 168

saturated fats 11, 18, 53, 54

Seligman, Martin 131, 176

Serotonin 77, 90, 91, 92, 207

SirT3 36

sleep i, 9, 11, 20, 23, 35, 36, 37, 38, 39, 40, 41, 42, 43, 44, 48, 50, 61, 62, 70, 76, 78, 80, 82, 83, 84, 91, 107, 111, 113, 115, 130, 203, 204, 205, 206, 207, 208

sound 26, 42, 43, 84, 152, 153, 155, 157, 158, 159, 168, 210

spinach 66, 68

stair walking 107

Stimulants 109

Stress 83, 99, 211

sucrose 55, 56

suprachiasmatic nuclei (SNC 48

Tart cherry juice 42

thalamus 156

The Center for Disease Control 57

tomatoes 42

Tracking 177

trans fats 53, 54, 104

Type 2 diabetes 55, 98

UCLA 102, 105

U-shaped curve 74, 76, 81, 83, 84, 94, 98, 100, 101, 103, 104, 106, 113, 115

Vasodilation 31

ventral medial prefrontal cortex 174

Visualization 141, 142

Vitamin C 67

Vitamin D 34

Vitamins C, D, and E 67, 68

walnuts 42

water 9, 13, 14, 20, 26, 27, 28, 30, 31, 70, 80, 92, 122, 142, 150, 206

Wernicke's area 155

working memory 29, 54, 100, 101, 103, 155, 157

Made in the USA
Monee, IL
03 December 2021